Neuropsychiatric
Movement Disorders

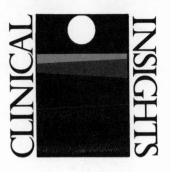

Neuropsychiatric Movement Disorders

Edited by
DILIP V. JESTE, M.D.
RICHARD JED WYATT, M.D.

Washington, D.C.

AMERICAN PSYCHIATRIC PRESS, INC.
Washington, D.C.

Library of Congress Cataloging in Publication Data

Main entry under title:

Neuropsychiatric movement disorders.

  (Clinical insights)
  Includes bibliographies.
  1. Movement disorders. 2. Neuropsychiatry.
I. Jeste, Dilip V. II. Wyatt, Richard Jed. III. Series.
[DNLM: 1. Movement Disorders. WL 390 N494]
RC925.5.N48   1984   616.7′4   84-14446
ISBN 0-88048-056-4 (pbk.)

Printed in the U.S.A.

Contents

Contributors

KENNETH J. BERGMANN, M.D.
Department of Neurology, The Mount Sinai School of Medicine, New York

DANIEL E. CASEY, M.D.
*Medical Research, Psychiatry and Neurology Services,
V.A. Medical Center, Portland, Ore.*

DONALD J. COHEN, M.D.
*Departments of Pediatrics, Psychiatry, and Psychology,
Yale University School of Medicine, New Haven, Conn.*

THOMAS E. HANSEN, M.D.
Department of Psychiatry, V.A. Medical Center, Portland, Ore.

DILIP V. JESTE, M.D.
*Adult Psychiatry Branch, National Institute of Mental Health,
Saint Elizabeths Hospital, Washington, D.C.*

JOHN M. KANE, M.D.
*Department of Psychiatry, Long Island–Jewish Hillside Hospital,
Glen Oaks, New York*

CRAIG N. KARSON, M.D.
*Adult Psychiatry Branch, National Institute of Mental Health,
Saint Elizabeths Hospital, Washington, D.C.*

BRUCE KINON, M.D.
Long Island–Jewish Hillside Hospital, Glen Oaks, New York

JAMES F. LECKMAN, M.D.
*Departments of Psychiatry and Pediatrics,
Yale University School of Medicine, New Haven, Conn.*

JEFFREY LIEBERMAN, M.D.
Long Island–Jewish Hillside Hospital, Glen Oaks, New York

SHARON ORT, R.N., M.P.H.
Clinical Nurse Specialist,
Yale University School of Medicine, New Haven, Conn.

MARK A. RIDDLE, M.D.
Departments of Psychiatry and Pediatrics,
University School of Medicine, New Haven, Conn.

BENNETT A. SHAYWITZ, M.D.
Departments of Pediatrics and Neurology,
Yale University School of Medicine, New Haven, Conn.

NANCY WEXLER, Ph.D.
Hereditary Disease Foundation, Beverly Hills, Calif.

MARGARET WOERNER, Ph.D.
Long Island–Jewish Hillside Hospital, Glen Oaks, New York

RICHARD JED WYATT, M.D.
Adult Psychiatry Branch, National Institute of Mental Health,
Saint Elizabeths Hospital, Washington, D.C.

MELVIN D. YAHR, M.D.
Department of Neurology, The Mount Sinai School of Medicine, New York

Preface

Any attempt to define the boundaries between psychiatry and neurology rigidly is unlikely to be successful. The great overlap between the two fields is well exemplified in the area of movement disorders. Most of the movement disorders seen clinically are neuropsychiatric in the true sense of the term. A study of these disorders clearly illustrates the fallacy of mind-body dichotomy.

Putting this book together has been an especially fruitful experience for us, thanks primarily to the high quality of the contributions. The task of editing a book is not always an unmixed blessing. One has to balance the need for some uniformity in style with the desirability of letting the contributors express themselves in their own unique fashion. Too rigid an approach is as unwelcome as an overly unstructured one. In the final analysis, however, it is the content of the chapters that determines the value of a book to the reader. The contributors to this volume, representing neurology, psychiatry, and psychology, made the editing of the book singularly pleasurable. We hope that clinicians, researchers, medical students, and paramedical professionals will find this book worthwhile.

Dilip V. Jeste, M.D.
Richard Jed Wyatt, M.D.

1

Parkinsonism and Its Treatment

Melvin D. Yahr, M.D.
Kenneth J. Bergmann, M.D.

1

Parkinsonism and Its Treatment

HISTORICAL PERSPECTIVE

In his essay on the "shaking palsy," James Parkinson in 1817 not only described the illness that now carries his name, but also alluded to its therapy. Though the treatments of the day were based on "little more than the evidence of inference" and consisted of bloodletting and blistering liniments, he wrote of paralysis agitans that "its real nature may be ascertained, and appropriate modes of relief, or even of cure, pointed out."

After this description of the parkinsonian triad (rigidity, bradykinesia, and tremor), a century passed before the morbid anatomy was described. Blocq and Marinesco (1893) first directed attention to the midbrain, reporting a case of hemiparkinsonism caused by a tuberculoma. F. H. Lewy (1913) described the round hyaline inclusion body that now bears his name, and in 1919 Tretiakoff described the cellular loss of the substantia nigra, now considered

Supported in part by grants NS 11631-11 from the National Institute of Neurological and Communicative Disorders and Stroke and RR-71 from the Division of Research Resources of the National Institutes of Health.

the sine qua non of classic parkinsonism (Yahr et al. 1972). The significance of the loss of pigmented neurons in the substantia nigra remained unknown until the demonstration by Ehringer and Hornykiewicz (1960) that striatal dopamine (DA) was lost in Parkinson's disease. Finally, with the development of histofluorescent neuron-mapping techniques, the projections of the substantia nigra and striatum have been documented (Fuxe et al. 1970).

Despite this hiatus, therapeutic intervention was limited only by the ingenuity of the patient's physician. The clinical efficacy of belladonna alkaloids derived from solanaceous plants was first formally noted over a century ago (Ordenstein 1867). By 1945, synthetic agents related to atropine and belladonna became available that had somewhat fewer peripheral antimuscarinic effects and consequently fewer of the myriad side effects that natural agents produce. With clarification of the biochemical pathology of parkinsonism came the first attempts to replace the lack of DA with L-dopa as its oral precursor (Birkmayer and Hornykiewicz 1961; Yahr et al. 1969). Over the last decade, it has become the gold standard against which all other therapies are now measured.

The "modern" era of pharmacotherapy dawned with expanded concepts of receptors, regulation of transmitter release, and transsynaptic alterations of neuronal systems that impinge upon the DA neuron. Though we are still far from understanding the cause of the illness and its relation to molecular pathology in the brain, the treatment of parkinsonism is no longer based on the unitary concept of restoring DA. Present-day pharmacotherapy is a result of a better understanding of what may be called the "parkinsonism syndrome," rather than a single disease process. The clinical illness may result from a loss of the nigral DA neurons or an interference with receptors in the striatum. Our thinking concerning the phenomenology of parkinsonism has also undergone evolution. Better treatments have resulted in clinical phenomena occurring in the illness that were not previously recognized. Whether these phenomena are related to progressive brain changes in patients who now live longer or are the effects of long-term therapy is debated. However, the recognition of all these current trends in neuroscience has enabled the development of a rational approach to therapy.

These advances have led to the development of neuropharmacological agents that mimic, stimulate, and regulate DA metabolism in the brain. They take advantage of these facts: L-dopa is decarboxylated to form DA; DA catabolism may be blocked by a monoamine oxidase inhibitor; DA receptors may be directly stimulated by synthetic agonists of DA; and agents active in other systems (e.g., anticholinergics) may also be used to alter the clinical symptomatology of the patient. These concepts and others form the cornerstone of therapy.

BASAL GANGLIA: CONNECTIONS AND FUNCTIONAL BIOCHEMISTRY

The extrapyramidal system is a loosely defined concept, the anatomical hub of which are the caudate nucleus and the putamen (the striatum, collectively), the globus pallidus or pallidum, and the substantia nigra (Brodal 1981). The striatum and pallidum (the basal ganglia) lie on the lateral aspect of the internal capsule, which separates them from the substantia nigra and other subthalamic nuclei. The striatum receives topographically arranged fibers from the cerebral cortex and the substantia nigra. In turn, the caudate and putamen project topographically upon the medial and lateral segments of the pallidum and the group of large, pigmented, DA-producing cells known as the "pars compacta" in the substantia nigra. This structure reciprocally innervates the striatum and pallidum. Nerve impulses converging upon the pallidum ultimately are received by the motor cortex by way of the thalamus, thus completing the circuit.

From a functional point of view, the most important neurotransmitters in the basal ganglia are acetylcholine, serotonin, γ-aminobutyric acid (GABA), and the monoamines DA and norepinephrine (NE). Though the exact role of each of these neurotransmitters has not been clarified, it is well established that acetylcholine and DA have a reciprocal relationship, with the former being excitatory and the latter inhibitory.

The precursor compounds and enzymes necessary for the production and degradation of acetylcholine and the catabolism of DA are found within the cellular substance of the basal ganglia. Experimental evidence demonstrates that DA is produced in the substantia nigra and is transported via a neuronal pathway, the nigrostriatal tract, to the caudate and putamen. There it has inhibitory actions, along with GABA, a putative inhibitory amino acid neurotransmitter. A homeostatic relationship is formed with acetylcholine, which exerts a net excitatory effect upon its striatal synapses, an effect antagonized by DA. Disturbance of this balance results in the myriad of phenomena ascribed to this area of the brain. In general, loss of DA results in excess cholinergic activity and is correlated with the slow, rigid parkinsonian symptom complex. Dopaminergic excess or cholinergic deficiency is thought to correlate with disorders of excessive and abnormal involuntary movements.

Therapy is undertaken with knowledge of the postulated relationships among DA, acetylcholine, and other regional transmitters.

PARKINSON'S DISEASE AND SYMPTOMATIC PARKINSONISM

When a patient has resting tremor, cogwheel rigidity, bradykinesia, paucity of movements with poor or unsustained initiation, impaired postural reflexes, hypomimia, seborrhea over the face, and drooling, the diagnosis of Parkinson's disease may be made with certainty. In one large series, 672 of 802 patients with parkinsonism were so designated (Hoehn and Yahr 1967).

It is important to note, however, that the majority of the symptoms and signs of parkinsonism—tremor, rigidity, and akinesia—may occur in a variety of disorders that affect the nervous system (Table 1).

Though idiopathic parkinsonism has a unique pathology well

Table 1 Parkinsonism

I. Primary (Idiopathic): Parkinson's Disease
II. Secondary (Symptomatic):
Infectious: Postviral encephalitis
Atherosclerotic
Drug-induced
Toxins: Carbon monoxide
Manganese
Metabolic: Parathyroid dysfunction
Anoxia
Miscellaneous:
Tumors
Head trauma
"Degenerative":
Parkinsonian dementia complex (Guam)
Striatonigral degeneration
Progressive supranuclear palsy
Olivopontocerebellar atrophies
Parkinsonism with autonomic dystrophy (Shy-Drager, multisystem atrophy)

suited to amelioration by oral replacement of a DA precursor, other illnesses may involve the striatum in a variety of ways. The basal ganglia and their connections may be affected by viral illnesses, system degenerations, stroke, and so forth, resulting in the clinical state of parkinsonism. These forms of symptomatic or "secondary" parkinsonism, may be accompanied by a varied constellation of other nervous system signs and symptoms. Their importance lies in the fact that both the neuron releasing the transmitter and the neuron with postsynaptic receptors must be intact in order for a neural circuit to be complete. Secondary parkinsonism is notable in that many forms respond only partially to levodopa therapy, often with drug-induced side effects. It is thought that these forms differ by having pathology not limited to one segment of motor circuitry (the DA neurons) as in classic parkinsonism.

Treatment of parkinsonism is lifelong, symptomatic, and supportive, the best program being the one tailored to the patient's needs and functional impairments. The aim of treatments is to keep the patient as functional as possible, running the gamut from psychotherapeutic intervention for the depression that frequently accompanies the illness to the introduction of new pharmacologic strategies.

Drug therapy follows certain practices derived empirically from the experience of treating parkinsonism. Patients commonly fall into three groups: the compensated patient early in the course, the decompensated patient, and the chronic, long-term patient who develops uneven and unpredictable responses to dopaminergic agents—the "on-off" syndrome.

There are differences between the effects of pharmacotherapy of Parkinson's disease and symptomatic parkinsonism: In the latter, expectations for the reversal of symptoms are fewer, and the nonextrapyramidal features remain resistant to antiparkinsonian agents.

Certain therapeutic considerations must be taken into account for particular ailments. Postencephalitic parkinsonism is remarkable for its responsiveness to anticholinergic agents and low tolerance for levodopa. The concern for treating the so-called "parkinson-plus syndromes" (parkinsonism in association with gaze palsies, autonomic dystrophy, dementia, or cerebellar incoordination) results from possible hazards owing to mobilizing a patient with poor judgment concerning motor function and increasing the chance of accidents. Treating the extrapyramidal syndrome of a patient with neuroleptic-induced parkinsonism may lull the physician into using higher doses of DA receptor blocking agents for longer periods of time, placing the patient at a higher risk for irreversible dyskinetic syndromes.

PHARMACOTHERAPY OF PARKINSON'S DISEASE

The early parkinsonian patient who is affected by a mild tremor in one extremity or a slight slowness and rigidity may require no treatment other than reassurance and encouragement to remain active. When progress is such that mild to moderate functional impairment begins, a number of medications are available (Table 2). The physiologic model best describing this situation is that of a person with substantial dopaminergic reserves in a low-function-

Table 2   Drugs Used in the Treatment of Parkinsonism

Generic Names	Trade Names	Dosage Form	Daily Dosage Range
Dopaminergics			
Levodopa (L-dopa)	Larodopa	250- and 500-mg caps and tabs	1–10 g
	Dopar	100-, 250-, and 500-mg caps	
Levodopa and carbidopa	Sinemet	10/100, 25/100, and 25/250 tabs	100/500–150/1500 mg
DA Receptor Agonists			
Bromocriptine	Parlodel	2.5- and 5-mg tabs and caps	20–100 mg
DA Catabolism Inhibitor			
L-Deprenil	Jumex L-Deprenalin	5-mg tabs	5–10 mg
DA-Releasing or Uptake Inhibitors			
Amantadine	Symmetrel	100-mg caps	100–300 mg
Imipramine	Tofranil	10-, 25-, and 50-mg tabs	30–150 mg
Amitriptyline	Elavil	10-, 25-, and 50-mg tabs	30–150 mg
Anticholinergics			
Hyoscine hydrobromide (scopolamine hydrobromide)	. . .	0.3-, 0.4-, and 0.6-mg tabs	1 tab 1–4 times daily
Benztropine mesylate	Cogentin	1- and 2-mg tabs parenteral solution (1 mg/2 cc vial)	1–6 mg 1 mg
Trihexyphenidyl	Artane	2- and 5-mg tabs 5-mg sustained-release caps	1–20 mg
	Tremin	2- and 5-mg tabs	
Cycrimine	Pagitane	1.25- and 2.5-mg tabs	1–20 mg
Procyclidine	Kemadrin	2- and 5-mg tabs	1–20 mg
Biperiden	Akineton	2-mg tabs 5-mg/ml parenteral solution	1–20 mg
Ethopropazine	Parsidol	10-, 50-, and 100-mg tabs	10–300 mg
Antihistamines			
Diphenhydramine	Benadryl	25- and 50-mg caps	25–200 mg
Orphenadrine HCl	Disipal	50-mg tabs	50–200 mg
Orphenadrine citrate	Norflex	100-mg tabs	100–200 mg
Chlorphenoxamine	Phenoxene	50-mg tabs	50–200 mg

NOTE.   DA = dopamine.

Table 3 Therapeutic Phases of Parkinson's Disease

Compensated (Stages 1 and 2)*
  Reassurance—No Pharmacological Agents
  Agents with CNS Antimuscarinic action
    Trihexyphenidyl
    Benztropine
    Diphenhydramine
  DA-Releasing or Reuptake-Inhibiting Agents
    Amantadine HCl
    Amphetamine (methamphetamine)
    Tricyclics (amitriptyline, imipramine)
  MAO-BI (Deprenyl)
Decompensated (Stages 3, 4, and 5*)
  Early
    Levodopa + PDI
    Levodopa + PDI = Anti-ACH
  Late
    Levodopa + PDI = MAO-BI (Deprenyl)
    DA receptor agonists
      Bromocriptine
      Pergolide
      Lisuride

NOTE. CNS = central nervous system; DA = dopamine; MAO-BI = monoamine oxidase-B inhibitor; PDI = peripheral decarboxylase inhibitor; ACH = acetylcholine.
  *Hoehn and Yahr scale (1967).

ing substantia nigra (Table 3). To rebalance cholinergic-dopaminergic relations, any one of the anticholinergic preparations may be used. These act to decrease the muscarinic effect of acetylcholine in the central nervous system (CNS), but have a peripheral action as well. The side effects caused by this peripheral action limit their dose and usefulness: dryness of the mouth and eyes, blurred vision, urinary retention (often exacerbating prostatism in men), and constipation. Mental aberrations of all forms, frequently hallucinatory or psychotic in nature, may occur, especially in the older patient.

An agent may be selected according to what degree of improvement is expected and how well side effects will be tolerated. Diphenhydramine (Benadryl) given 50–100 mg/day in three or four divided doses will yield only moderate improvement but with fewer side effects, mostly drowsiness. It may be increased to 200 mg/day as needed. The piperidyl family of drugs, of which trihexyphenidyl (Artane) is most popular, is more potent. Two milligrams three times a day is a good beginning, but even at this dose we have witnessed untoward mental effects, especially in the older, demented patient. However, most patients are able to tolerate up to 10 mg/day and occasionally more.

Benztropine mesylate (Cogentin) of the tropane family closely mimics atropine and often produces intolerable side effects before reaching its full therapeutic level. As such, it is often useful to combine it with other medications as adjunctive therapy. It acts over a longer period of time, and 1 or 2 mg at bedtime is helpful for the patient whose sleep is disturbed by lying in one position all night or who has trouble upon arising in the morning. Of the many anticholinergic agents available to the physician, the choice may be best dictated by familiarity with just a few of them.

Amantadine (Symmetrel), originally used for influenza prophylaxis in the elderly, was serendipitously found to aid parkinsonism. Its mechanism is unclear. Given 100 mg two or three times a day, the patient will note some improvement in 2 or 3 days. It may safely be combined with other agents. However, as with most dopaminergic agents, its best effect occurs within the first 3–4 months of use, decreasing thereafter to a state of lower efficacy. Its major adverse effects are confusion and hallucinatory states, chronic dependent edema, and livedo reticularis, a skin discoloration that may be permanent.

The decompensated parkinsonian patient has theoretically used up his or her nigral DA stores and requires a replacement to act upon striatal receptor sites (Table 3). The efficacy of levodopa as a precursor to DA is well documented (Yahr et al. 1969). When previously used, a certain amount would be converted to DA outside the nervous system by dopa decarboxylase, its ubiquitous anabolic enzyme. DA outside the CNS causes unpleasant side effects: nausea, gastric upset, cardiac dysrhythmias, and hypotension. By concomitantly giving carbidopa or benserazide, peripheral decarboxylase inhibitors unable to cross the blood-brain barrier (Sinemet and Madopar, respectively), L-dopa is selectively used within the CNS, yielding a minimum of side effects, with a fourth of the L-dopa that one would need otherwise.

Although side effects are few with a levodopa/carbidopa combination, it should be used judiciously in the patient with a history of cerebrovascular or cardiovascular ailments or affective or psychotic disorders. The presence of hemolytic disorders of glucose-6-phosphate dehydrogenase deficiency contraindicates its use. Vitamins containing pyridoxine (B6) should be discontinued. Monoamine oxidase inhibitors may potentiate its effects.

When starting therapy, various combinations of carbidopa/levodopa are available: 10/100, 25/100, 25/250 (the numerator referring to milligrams of carbidopa, the denominator to milligrams of levodopa). In an average person, it takes approximately 75–150 mg/day carbidopa to fully inhibit peripheral dopa decarboxylase and resultant side effects. Thus, any combination of pills may be chosen to achieve this. Treatment is best begun at a low dose: 10/100 or 25/100 three times a day, increased by one tablet every third day. Generally some response is seen when the patient is receiving 50/500 per day. Rarely, at this dose, some patients are sensitive to the levodopa being insufficiently blocked peripherally; changing to 25/100-mg pills or adding carbidopa by itself to the regimen often alleviates this while supplying the same amount of levodopa. The goal of a minimum dosage achieving a tolerable degree of function generally is reached at 70/700–100/1,000 daily. An occasional patient requires up to 150/1,500 per day, and fully 5 percent of patients with Parkinson's disease as well as the parkinsonism-plus syndromes may not respond. In our experience, the patient is left with some residual dysfunction, but chasing this with increasing amounts of levodopa is ineffective and often brings out troublesome dyskinesias. After the necessary daily amount of medication is reached, it is attempted to integrate it into the patient's daily life with three or four divided doses. Often, as time passes and the illness progresses, more frequent scheduling is required.

There is some evidence that the efficacy of levodopa attenuates after several years (Yahr 1976). Among our parkinsonian patients, each year of therapy brings an additional proportion who respond less well, requiring more frequent and larger doses, or who develop paradoxical responses to therapy. Such responses include sudden switches from a dyskinetic state with choreoathetotic and dystonic features to a severely frozen rigid state (on-off phenomena). The basis for this is unknown. Because of this problem, we attempt to manage parkinsonism with adjunctive agents for as long as possible prior to beginning levodopa. Naturally, there are reasons to deviate from this: a patient requiring an unusual degree of agility, proximity to retirement, social reasons for concealing the illness, and so forth.

Patients are generally well maintained at a given level of Sinemet, continuing to improve slowly even after the steady state is reached. After a period of time, 2–4 years on average, the patient experiences a falling off in the effect. This first occurs at the end of a dosing period prior to the next pill. The solution is to shorten the interval between doses while maintaining the same total daily amount. Occasionally, additional levodopa is required. Eventually such a diminution in effect (off-period) occurs without pattern, often with such rapidity that a patient may literally be frozen in midstep. Concurrently, the on-period, during which the medication has beneficial effects, reverses the parkinsonism in an extreme fashion, associated with hypotonia and dyskinesias. These may affect any and all parts of the body and may be incapacitating. In most, however, on-periods are preferred, especially if mild, owing to increased mobility. Early on, dyskinesias at the start of the dose period may be associated with a failure of the dose to last through the entire interval; this may similarly be corrected by smaller, more frequent medication intervals. As with the off-period, this eventually appears unrelated to the dosing interval.

The chronic parkinsonian patient, troubled by severe on-off phenomena, remains the most difficult patient to care for. Attempts to establish the best intervals and dose of levodopa may take weeks, aggravated by occasionally seeing an excellent response one day and chaos the next. Having patients keep a daily diary of the number of on-periods and their duration is a help in documenting their response. With the idea that fluctuating levels of levodopa or progressive deterioration in the functional biochemistry of the striatum may be at the bottom of this difficulty, a number of agents have been developed as adjuncts to dopaminergic therapy. In general, they have longer half-lives than levodopa and have the effect of increasing the availability of DA at the synapse by increasing its release, inhibiting its breakdown, or stimulating its receptors directly.

Bromocriptine (Parlodel), a semisynthetic ergot derivative first used in the galactorrhea-amenorrhea syndrome, acts both pre- and postsynaptically as a DA receptor agonist. Although not as effective as DA alone, it is useful in smoothing out the medication effect, producing less fluctuation in the clinical state when on-off phenomena are troublesome. It may become less effective after the initial several months of therapy. While common side effects include nausea, hypotension, and additional dyskinesia, the most troublesome is the production of mental aberrations and hallucinosis at therapeutic levels. Bromocriptine is begun at low doses, generally ≤7.5 mg in three divided doses, and increased slowly every few days. A response is generally noted at 20 mg/day but becomes optimal at the 30- to 50-mg/day level. Other synthetic ergot derivatives (lisuride and pergolide) are under investigation. The outcome remains unclear, but pergolide has been helpful in our hands with a relative paucity of side effects.

Deprenyl, a selective monoamine oxidase-B inhibitor, increases DA at the synaptic cleft by inhibiting its catabolic enzyme. It too is under investigation and not yet released for general use in the United States though available in Europe. Tricyclic antidepressants in general are somewhat anticholinergic. Useful in treating both the common attendant depression of parkinsonism and the movement disorder itself, they have relatively few serious side effects. Imipramine (Tofranil) or amitriptyline (Elavil) may be given at 25 mg three or four times per day.

For the patient with severe difficulties, other measures may be needed. Occasionally, it is beneficial to take the patient off all dopaminergic medication during a hospitalization for a "drug holiday." Often when restarting therapy 7-10 days later, better management is attained with smaller doses at a more frequent schedule. Unfortunately, this effect is usually short lived. Care must be taken to avoid a parkinsonian crisis in the patient with severe bulbar manifestations, who will then be threatened with aspiration and inanition. We have found the severe rigidity attendant to drug holidays to be of great concern and terrible anxiety to the patient who has often not realized the extent to which the disease has progressed.

A helpful and sympathetic approach to the plight of the patient aids the acceptance of the present limitations to therapy posed by parkinsonism. As investigation in this field progresses, it is hoped that newer agents and strategies for their use will yield the success that levodopa has for the majority of those afflicted.

FUTURE TRENDS

It is becoming increasingly recognized that despite replacement therapy of depleted neurotransmitters in Parkinson's disease, the illness progresses inexorably. The exact mechanism(s) are poorly defined but at least include a loss of trophic factors when actual nerve cells denervate their target structures. Transsynaptic alterations of receptor systems are well documented and have led to the approach of attempting pharmacologically to stimulate the next cell in the neuronal network of structures related to movement. A few such agents are presently under investigation.

Paradoxical akinesia, a difficult symptom to treat in parkinsonism, manifests itself by difficulty in initiating walking. Thus, the patient frequently falls, often resulting in hip fractures and other severe disabilities. This "freezing" phenomenon may be identified as an independent sign, after other features of parkinsonism with which it is intimately intertwined have been well controlled with L-dopa. It may also appear as an early characteristic of Parkinson's disease in the so-called "pure akinetic form" not accompanied by significant degrees of tremor and rigidity. At present, there is little knowledge about the neurophysiological mechanisms underlying this phenomenon, but it has been suggested the the lowering of NE in the CNS as a result of degeneration of the locus ceruleus is responsible (Nagatsu et al. 1979).

Preliminary reports suggest that D,L-threo-dihydroxyphenylserine, a precursor of NE decarboxylated by aromatic amino acid decarboxylase to form NE directly (thus bypassing DA in the biosynthetic pathway) may be successfully used to alleviate this disturbing symptom (Narabayashi et al. 1984).

GABA and DA appear to have an intimately associated modulatory action upon each other. The nigrostriatal DA pathway comes under feedback control via a GABA-mediated striatonigral pathway. Outflow pathways from the pallidum and the substantia nigra to lower motor structures are also thought to utilize GABA as a neurotransmitter. Few, if any, centrally active agents capable of enhancing the action of this neurotransmitter in the brain have been available. Recently, progabide, a new postsynaptic agonist, has been developed, and preliminary trials suggest that it acts in a way traditionally considered "dopaminergic" (Bergmann et al. 1984). At least in patients with on-off phenomena, it lessens the severity of parkinsonian periods and increases the amount of functional time during the waking hours.

Whether these agents or others become important adjuncts to current antiparkinson therapy remains to be seen.

More physiological approaches toward supplying missing factors to the parkinsonian patient have been received with great interest. Following the lead from animal work using fetal tissues as grafts to DA-denervated host rat brains, investigators have developed techniques to ascertain that functional brain transplants with intact synaptic connections are possible. The first two human transplants using adrenal tissue autografts have been performed in Sweden, but it is clearly premature to evaluate the future of this technique.

Other investigators are looking into the etiology of the cellular damage in parkinsonism. Work with 6-hydroxydopamine, which is toxic to monoamine cells (Cohen 1983), and N-methyl-4-phenyl-1,2,3,6-tetrahydropyridine (NMPTD), which causes selective nigral damage, will, it is hoped, provide clues as to the susceptibility of this population of cells to damage by intrinsic and environmental factors. With the early detection of parkinsonism and prevention of further cellular loss, Parkinson's dream of a cure for his disease may come to pass.

References

Bergmann KJ, Limongi JCP, Lowe Y-H, et al: Progabide in decompensated Parkinson's disease: implications of dopaminergic-GABAergic interactions for levodopa-induced fluctuations, in Catecholamines, vol C. Edited by Usden E, Carlsson A. New York, Liss (in press)

Birkmayer W, Hornykiewicz O: Der L-Dioxyphenylalanin (=LDopa) Effeckt bei der Parkinson Akinese. Wien Klin Wochenschr 73:787–788, 1961

Blocq P, Marinesco G: Sur un cas de tremblement parkinsonien hemiplegique symptomatique d'une tumeur du pedoncule cerebral. C R Soc Biol (Paris) 5:105–111, 1893

Brodal A: Neurological Anatomy in Relation to Clinical Medicine. New York, Oxford, 1981

Cohen G: The pathobiology of Parkinson's disease: biochemical aspects of dopamine neuron senescence. J Neural Transm 19 (Suppl): 89–103, 1983

Ehringer H, Hornykiewicz O: Verteiluing von Noradrenalin und Dopamin (3 Hydroxytyramin) im Gehirn des Menschen und ihr Verhalten bei Erkrankungen des Extrapyramidalen Systems. Klin Wochenschr 38:1236–1239, 1960

Fuxe K, Hokfelt T, Ungerstadt U: Morphological and functional aspects of central monoamine neurons. Int Rev Neurobiol 13:93–126, 1970

Hoehn MM, Yahr MD: Parkinsonism: onset, progression, and mortality. Neurology 17:427–442, 1967

Lewy FH: Zur pathologischen anatomie der paralysis agitans. Deutscha Zeitschrift für Nervenheilkunde 50:50–55, 1913

Nagatsu T, Kato T, Nagatsu I, et al: Catecholamine-related enzymes in the brains of patients with parkinsonism and Wilson's disease. Adv Neurol 24:283–292, 1979

Narabayashi H, Kondo T, Nagatsu T, et al: L-Threo-3,4-dihydroxy-phenylserine (L-Threo-DOPS) for freezing symptom in parkinsonism. Adv Neurol 40:497–503, 1984

Ordenstein L: Sur la Paralysie Agitante. Paris, Martinet, 1867, p 32

Parkinson J: An Essay on the Shaking Palsy. London, Whittingham and Rowland, 1817

Tretiakoff D: Contribution a l'etude de l'anatomie pathologique du locus niger de Soemmering (Thesis: Paris, 1919). Cited in Greenfield JG: The pathology of Parkinson's disease, in James Parkinson. Edited by Critchley M. London, Macmillan, 1955

Yahr MD: Evaluation of long term therapy in Parkinson's disease: mortality and therapeutic efficacy, in Advances in Parkinsonism. Edited by Birkmayer W, Hornykiewicz O. Basle, Roche, 1976, pp 435–443

Yahr MD, Duvoisin RC, Schear MJ, et al: Treatment of parkinsonism with levodopa. Arch Neurol 21:343–354, 1969

Yahr MD, Wolf A, Antunes J-L, et al: Autopsy findings in parkinsonism following treatment with levodopa. Neurology 22:56–71, 1972

2

Tourette's Syndrome

Donald J. Cohen, M.D.
Mark A. Riddle, M.D.
James F. Leckman, M.D.
Sharon Ort, R.N., M.P.H.
Bennett A. Shaywitz, M.D.

2

Tourette's Syndrome

DIAGNOSTIC CRITERIA

Tics are rapid, repetitive, purposeless, involuntary movements of functionally related muscle groups that are more easily recognized than precisely defined. Age at onset, duration of symptoms, and the presence of vocal or phonic tics in addition to motor tics are generally used to divide tic disorders into different diagnostic categories.

A common disorder of childhood, transient tic disorder is characterized by one or more simple motor tics that wax and wane in severity over a period of weeks to months. Eye blinking or other facial tics are often seen; less frequently, simple phonic tics (e.g., sniffing, throat clearing, or noises) are observed. The tic(s) can be voluntarily suppressed for brief periods of time, or exacerbated by stress, excitement, or fatigue. Although adequate epidemiological studies are lacking, prevalence estimates for transient tic disorder range as high as 15 percent of all school age children. By

This research was supported by The Gateposts Foundation, Mental Health Clinical Research Center grant MH 30929, NICHD grant HD 03008, and the John Merck Fund.

definition, transient tic disorder does not persist for >1 year. However, simple transient tics may return after a period of remission. This disorder is usually mild, aggregates in families, and does not interfere with school performance or peer relationships.

Chronic motor tic disorder is differentiated from the transient disorder by its duration of >1 year and by the relatively unchanging character of the tics over time. This is probably a heterogeneous diagnostic category with some forms being closely related to Tourette's syndrome (TS). Age at onset varies; some patients do not develop symptoms until adulthood.

TS, the most debilitating of the tic disorders, is characterized by multiform, frequently changing motor and phonic tics and a range of behavioral symptoms. Prevailing diagnostic criteria include: age at onset between 2 and 15 years; rapid, recurrent, repetitive, purposeless, involuntary movements affecting multiple muscle groups; multiple vocal tics; ability to suppress movements voluntarily for minutes to hours; variations in the intensity of the symptoms over weeks or months; and duration of >1 year (American Psychiatric Association 1980). Although these criteria may be operationally sound in practice, emerging clinical research supports the need for refinements regarding age at onset, the "involuntary" character of the tics, and the full range of associated behavioral symptoms (Cohen et al. 1982).

HISTORY

The 1489 description of a priest with motor and phonic tics, in an inquisitional tract on methods of detecting and treating witches possessed by the devil, was the first recorded account of a person with possible TS. In 1885 George Gilles de la Tourette published a report in which he described the syndrome that bears his name. Although it is difficult to capture the clinically rich and clear quality of his report in a single paragraph, the following quotation summarizes Gilles de la Tourette's conceptualization of the disorder (Goetz and Klawans 1982):

Let us recall first some of the fundamental symptoms: 1) this illness is hereditary; it is characterized by motor incoordination in the form of abrupt muscular jerks that are often severe enough to make the patient jump; 2) the incoordination can be accompanied by articulated or inarticulated sounds. When articulated, the words are often repetitions of words which the patient may have just heard. Such vocal imitation (echolalia) may have a physical corollary whereby the subject imitates an act or gesture that he has just seen; 3) among the expressions which the patient may repeatedly utter during one of his convulsions, some have the special character of being obscene (coprolalia); 4) the physical and mental health of these patients is otherwise basically normal. The condition seems incurable and life long, with onset in childhood.

Interest in TS increased dramatically in the 1960s with the emergence of successful pharmacological treatments (Shapiro et al. 1978). Currently, multiple disciplines are studying TS in order to define the relationships among the behavioral, genetic, and neurochemical characteristics of the disorder. Many investigators consider TS to be a model for neuropsychiatric disorders with childhood onset: There appear to be a genetically determined biological vulnerability, an age-dependent expression of symptoms that may be related to central nervous system (CNS) ontogeny, sexual dimorphism, and environmental stress-dependent fluctuations in symptomatic severity (Leckman et al. 1984).

CLINICAL FEATURES AND DIAGNOSIS

Clinical Expression

The motor and phonic tics of TS can be characterized by their frequency, complexity, and the degree to which they disrupt the patient's ongoing activities and daily life. Simple motor tics are fast, darting, repetitive, meaningless muscular events—contractions of functionally related muscle groups. Examples include eye blinking, facial grimacing, nose twitching, shoulder shrugs, head or arm jerks, finger movements, jaw snaps, and the rapid jerking of any part of the body. Complex motor tics are usually slower and more purposeful in appearance. They can involve any type of movement the body can produce, including touching, kicking, hopping, throwing, and clapping, as well as gyrating, writhing movements and "dystonic" posturing. Often the patient will attempt to "camouflage" these movements. Repetitive grooming behaviors, such as brushing hair away from the face, are common examples of camouflaging. Complex motor tics may become very organized, ritualistic, and "compulsive" in character. The need to stand up repeatedly and move a piece of furniture into "just the right position" or to arrange objects neatly is compulsive in character. Occasionally, patients develop self-abusive behaviors such as biting, head banging, or eye poking.

Linguistically meaningless noises and sounds, such as coughing, sniffling, spitting, barking, grunting, and hissing, typify simple phonic tics. Complex phonic tics involve sudden ejaculation of inappropriate words or phrases, e.g., "Oops!" "Yup, you got it," or "Now, now, now. . . . " Patients may also change the flow of speech by slurring a phrase, altering volume and/or pitch, or mimicking the speech of others.

Coprolalia, the sudden utterance of obscenities, is the most socially distressing complex phonic symptom. Initially manifested by the abrupt utterance of first syllables (e.g., "fff, ffuu" or "sh, sh, shi") or single obscene words, this symptom may progress to more elaborate forms in which the swearing is embedded in longer statements and may take the form of sexual, hostile, or insulting statements (e.g., "Nice tits!" or "I love you, I hate you"). Coprolalic symptoms are experienced as "ego dystonic" or "ego alien" even by patients who are generally impulsive or labile.

Associated Disorders

In addition to the motor and phonic symptoms, several behavioral symptoms are often seen in patients with TS, including diminished ability to concentrate, impulsiveness, impaired regulation of activity, and disabling obsessions and compulsions.

As many as 50 percent of children with TS satisfy the diagnostic criteria for attention deficit disorder (ADD; inattentiveness and impulsivity) and hyperactivity. The onset of the ADD and hyperactivity often precedes the onset of tics. Although most TS patients do not have primary learning disabilities, the ADD and hyperactivity can substantially impair school performance. Attentional problems persist during periods of tic remission and usually continue into adulthood. Other problems affecting school or work performance are trouble in completing work, peer relationship difficulties, and graphomotor impairments. In a sizable proportior of TS patients, specific learning disabilities are also present.

The obsessive-compulsive symptoms seen in patients with TS usually appear late in the developmental course of the syndrome. These symptoms, such as obsessive doubting about a decision or elaborate compulsive rituals involving complicated mimicking, may be severely disabling.

Phenomenology

There is a wide range of symptomatology and impairment seen in patients with TS. In its most severe forms, patients may have almost constant, uncountable motor and phonic tics, paroxysms of full-body movements, shouting, and self-abusive behavior. Milder forms may present with only a few tics per minute or hour.

For the individual patient, the frequency, severity, and mixture of symptoms may vary markedly over short and long periods of time and are place and state dependent. The bewildering waxing and waning of symptoms complicates diagnostic and therapeutic efforts—patients may "lose" their tics when they enter the doctor's office. Furthermore, tics may be inhibited in school but become nonstop as soon as the child arrives at home; or be quiescent during focused activity but exacerbate while relaxing in front of the television. Although rigorous data are lacking, life events and stresses seem frequently to precede symptomatic exacerbations.

The tics of patients with TS are currently defined as "involun-tary." This definition is consistent with the reported inner experi-ence of many, especially younger, patients with TS. However, some children and many adult patients describe antecedent, fleeting sensory "signals" or "urges," suggesting the possible involvement of sensory systems as well as motor pathways (Bliss et al. 1980). Patients may feel an increasing tension localized to a part of the body or throat; the tension will mount, along with a sense of anxiety; finally, the patients will feel that they will explode unless they perform a tic or emit a sound. Following the discharge, a refractory period of reduced tension may be followed by a progressive increase in tension either at the same site or in some other part of the body. Some patients report "attending to" these inner signals in order to prevent or modify the occurrence of a tic. This ability to modify or inhibit tics calls into question their characterization as involuntary.

Natural History

For the typical patient with TS, attentional problems, impulsivity, and hyperactivity emerge during the late preschool years (see Figure 1). These symptoms usually precede tics or develop concurrently with a few simple ones. More persistent motor and phonic tics occur later; the mean age at onset of motor tics is 7 years, with a range of from 2 to 18 years, whereas the mean age at onset of phonic tics is 11 years. Often progressing in a rostro-caudal pattern, simple motor tics are usually followed by complex motor tics. Phonic symptoms develop after the motor symptoms. The severest and most disabling symptoms (e.g., rituals, compulsions, graphic descriptions of sexual or aggressive acts) tend to present last. There are many exceptions to this typical description such as the rapid emergence of symptoms over a brief interval of time or the onset of phonic tics prior to motor tics.

Clinical experience suggests that the most severely afflicted patients have the earliest age at onset and the severest early behavioral and attentional symptoms. Although adequate data are lacking on the natural history of such patients, at least some develop long-term or even permanent remissions of their motor and phonic tics. In some cases, obsessive and compulsive symp-

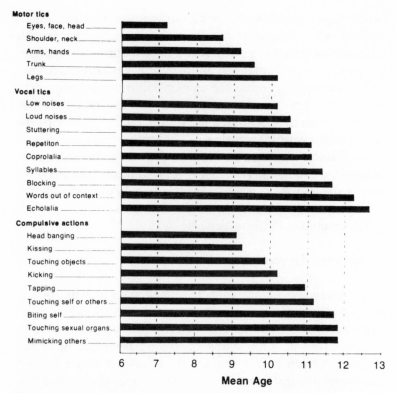

Figure 1 Mean age at occurrence of Tourette tics. Reproduced with permission from Jagger et al. (1982).

toms may be the sole or major remaining symptoms. Typically, however, TS patients continue to have motor and phonic tics intermittently throughout life.

Differential Diagnosis

The differential diagnosis of tics includes choreiform, dystonic, athetoid, myoclonic, and hemiballismic movements. In addition, spasms, synkinesis, and dyskinesias may be difficult to distinguish from tics.

Because of the increased recognition of TS in recent years, a patient with moderate to severe symptoms is unlikely to be misdiagnosed. However, it may be difficult to differentiate a child with severe ADD and hyperactivity from one with the early manifestations of TS. In addition, patients with amphetamine intoxication, cerebrovascular accident, Lesch-Nyhan syndrome, Wilson's disease, Sydenham's and Huntington's chorea, multiple sclerosis, schizophrenia, general paresis, and organic mental disorders may present with abnormal movements. However, these disorders can be distinguished from TS by clinical evaluation (e.g., none of these disorders include phonic tics) and appropriate laboratory tests. In practice, careful history taking and observation provide the diagnosis since no other disorder mimics the full TS.

Prognosis

The long-term outcome for patients with TS ranges from complete remission of symptoms to severe debilitation that can require intermittent institutionalization. Ultimate social adaptation probably depends more upon behavioral and attentional symptoms than on motor or phonic tics. Factors affecting outcome include intelligence, attentional problems, school achievement, the family's response to the illness, the severity of the motor and phonic symptoms, and the patient's response to medication and/or other therapeutic interventions.

EPIDEMIOLOGY/GENETICS

TS occurs in all major racial groups and appears to have a stable pattern of clinical expression across cultures. Until recently, TS was thought to be a rare disorder. However, with increasing medical recognition and public awareness, many more patients with TS are being diagnosed. Although definitive epidemiological studies are lacking, estimates of lifetime prevalence range from 4 to 10 per 10,000. Based on known cases in Connecticut, we have estimated that the prevalence of full-blown TS is at least 5 per 10,000 (i.e., somewhat higher than autism). Two very recent lines of evidence suggest that the prevalence of TS may be even higher. Genetic evidence suggests that TS and multiple tics aggregate in families and are on the same spectrum (Pauls et al. 1981). Although preliminary, these data would increase the prevalence of the TS diathesis to perhaps 50 per 10,000.

Most epidemiological evidence regarding TS has been derived from family history data. Investigators have recently shown that the use of structured interviews in addition to family history information may increase the identification of chronic multiple tics and TS severalfold (Pauls et al. 1984).

Boys are more commonly affected than girls. Estimates of the sex ratio (male:female) vary from 3:1 to 9:1. Girls may require a stronger genetic predisposition (i.e., more affected individuals in their family) before expressing the disorder.

TS may be genetically associated with other neuropsychiatric disorders, particularly ADD and obsessive-compulsive disorder (see Chapter 4). Further genetic and biological studies are necessary to establish the precise nature of the relationship between TS and other disorders.

ETIOLOGY/PATHOGENESIS

Although both hereditary and environmental factors have been implicated, the etiology and pathogenesis of TS have not been established.

Genetics

The previous section reviewed data suggesting some form of vertical transmission of TS, the close relationship between TS and transient and chronic tic disorders, and the sex threshold effect (i.e., although boys are more commonly affected with TS than girls, the relatives of girls with TS are at a greater risk for TS or chronic tic disorders than are the relatives of boys with TS; Pauls et al. 1981).

Anecdotal case reports of twins indicate a very high concordance rate for monozygotic twins for TS, in the range of 75–95 percent. In contrast, the results from a recent questionnaire study of 30 monozygotic twin pairs in which at least one twin had TS indicated only a 53 percent concordance for TS and a 76 percent concordance for TS or another tic disorder (Price et al. unpublished data). Concordant twin pairs were also frequently found to show differing levels in the severity of symptom expression. These more recent data provide support for the importance of environmental (nongenetic) factors in the expression of TS.

Although genetic factors appear to exert a powerful influence on the etiology of TS, they are not found in all patients. Even if the gene(s) underlying the disorder are identified, it will be necessary to explicate their molecular mode of action and to identify specific risk factors that may cause this vulnerability to be expressed.

Environment

The onset of TS symptoms and the transitional periods that occur in its waxing and waning course often seem unrelated to environmental factors. However, clinical experience and pilot epidemiological studies indicate that periods of increased anxiety and emotional stress are regularly accompanied by an exacerbation of TS symptoms (Jagger et al. 1982).

A second environmental (nongenetic) factor known to exacerbate TS symptoms is exposure to stimulant medication. Recently, investigators have reported several series of patients whose use of stimulants (e.g., methylphenidate, dextroamphetamine, and pemoline) correlated with the onset of motor and phonic tics. Stimulant medications can produce complex stereotypies in animals that disappear when the stimulants are terminated; similarly, some children treated with stimulant medication develop simple motor tics (such as eye blinking or mouth puckering) that disappear with reduction or cessation of the medication. It is more controversial whether stimulants can actually trigger or induce prolonged TS or chronic multiple tics that persist following the termination of medication. However, cases have been reported in which this seems to have occurred (Golden 1974; Lowe et al. 1982). The most convincing clinical evidence may come from ticfree children who received two courses of stimulant medication. During the first course, tics appeared after months of treatment and stopped with drug termination; during the second course, tics appeared within days and persisted for months or continuously when stimulants were withdrawn. These children seemed to have had TS "kindled" by repeated exposure to stimulants. A complication in this story is that some children—but, importantly, not all—who had TS emerge during the course of stimulant treatment had a family history of TS or tics and perhaps were genetically vulnerable. Further, it is not possible to know whether a subgroup of children with ADD who developed TS while taking stimulants were already on their way to developing this disorder anyway. Detailed neurochemical and genetic studies will be needed to tease out the interacting factors involved in the induction and exacerbation of tics and TS by stimulants.

Neurochemistry

Although several neurochemical systems have been implicated in the pathogenesis of TS, the most convincing evidence supports the role of dopaminergic systems. Clinical pharmacological evidence includes: the dramatic suppression of tics by dopamine (DA) receptor-blocking agents (e.g., haloperidol, pimozide); the emergence of TS-like symptoms in psychiatric patients following the withdrawal of neuroleptics (i.e., DA receptor blockers); the symptomatic exacerbations produced by stimulant medications (direct DA agonists); and the amelioration of TS symptoms by DA autoreceptor stimulants (e.g., apomorphine, piribedil; Feinberg and Carroll 1979). Neurochemical evidence includes lowered levels of cerebrospinal fluid (CSF) homovanillic acid (HVA; the principal metabolite of central DA) in many TS patients (Butler et al. 1979; Cohen et al. 1979). A "supersensitive" DA receptor, with subsequent negative feedback to the presynaptic dopaminergic neuron, is one hypothesis that could explain these findings (Friedhoff 1982).

The evidence for noradrenergic involvement in the pathogenesis of TS also comes primarily from clinical pharmacological studies. Clonidine, an imidazoline derivative that preferentially stimulates α_2-adrenergic receptors probably located presynaptically, is effective in reducing the symptoms of TS in many patients. Stimulation of these α_2-receptors results in a decreased release of norepinephrine (NE) at the synapse. Studies using microiontophoretic techniques have shown that clonidine inhibits the spontaneous firing of the locus ceruleus (the primary site of noradrenergic cell bodies in brain) and reduces brain NE turnover. Clonidine also acutely lowers the concentration of plasma free 3-methoxy-4-hydroxyphenethylglycol (MHPG; the principal central metabolite of NE; Leckman et al. 1980, 1981). However, there are several observations that raise questions about the role of NE in the pathogenesis of TS. First, clonidine is effective in ameliorating the symptoms of opiate withdrawal in addicted newborn infants (Hoder et al. 1981); yet studies in rat pups have shown that α_2-adrenergic receptors are not functional until ≥ 21 days of age, suggesting that clonidine may have other mechanisms of action. Second, our studies of CSF and urine MHPG, and plasma NE in TS patients have not generally revealed differences from normal controls.

The mode of action of clonidine in TS may involve indirect effects on the dopaminergic system as evidenced by elevated levels of plasma HVA following chronic clonidine treatment (Leckman et al. 1983). The report that a positive clinical response to haloperidol during a double-blind crossover trial predicted a positive response to clonidine is also consistent with this hypothesis (Borison et al. 1982). In addition, results from animal studies indicate that noradrenergic activity can alter DA-mediated activity (Antelman and Caggiula 1977). Interestingly, serotonergic mechanisms have been suggested as the link between central noradrenergic and dopaminergic ones (Bunney and DeReimer 1982).

There is currently insufficient evidence to support a hypothesis of direct serotonergic involvement in the pathogenesis of TS. Medications that act by increasing or decreasing serotonergic activity do not consistently affect TS symptoms. However, studies of CSF 5-hydroxyindoleacetic acid (the principal central metabolite of serotonin) in TS patients have tended to reveal differences from normal controls, with TS patients showing lowered concentrations.

Although the data are limited and contradictory, cholinergic systems have also been implicated in the pathogenesis of TS. Clinical pharmacological evidence generally suggests that cholinergic agents (e.g., physostigmine, deanol, choline, and lecithin) reduce TS symptoms, whereas anticholinergic agents (e.g., scopolamine) exacerbate them, supporting an acetylcholine deficiency hypothesis (Stahl and Berger 1982). In addition, elevated red blood cell choline was found in TS patients and their relatives; however, the relationship of this finding to brain cholinergic function is unclear (Hanin et al. 1979).

It is possible that the expression of TS involves several neurotransmitter systems operating in a cascading or reinforcing manner. Various aspects of the disorder may involve different neurotransmitters or a balance between them. For example, motor symptoms may express dopaminergic overactivity, whereas difficulties with inhibition (e.g., distractibility, coprolalia) may represent the engagement of noradrenergic or serotonergic mechanisms. It is likely that other neurotransmitter systems (e.g., neuropeptide, GABAergic) will be implicated in the future.

Neurophysiology and Neuropsychology

The electroencephalogram (EEG), computed tomography (CT) scan, sensory and visual evoked response, premovement EEG potential, and neuropsychological test battery have been employed in the study of TS.

Numerous investigators have reported abnormal EEGs in 35–65 percent of subjects with TS. This high incidence of EEG abnormalities has been interpreted to indicate anatomical dysfunction. Nonlocalized sharp waves and/or slowing are most frequently observed; epileptiform activity is uncommon. One study found that TS patients with abnormal EEGs were more likely to have other objective signs of neurological dysfunction or were taking haloperidol, a drug known to disturb the EEG (Bergen et al. 1982). We have found that TS patients with abnormal EEGs have a significantly younger age at onset (Volkmar et al. 1984). Otherwise, the EEG does not appear to be of either clinical or prognostic significance.

We found that 6 (37 percent) of 16 subjects with TS had mildly to markedly abnormal CT scans (Caparulo et al. 1981). The most common abnormality was ventricular dilation. Four (67 percent) of the 6 subjects with abnormal CT scans also had abnormal EEGs, whereas only 1 (10 percent) of the 10 children with a normal CT scan had an abnormal EEG. No localized CT findings have been reported in patients with TS.

Preliminary studies of cortical somatosensory evoked potentials in patients with TS revealed no abnormalities (Obeso et al. 1982), whereas visually evoked responses showed wave IV amplitude changes (Domino et al. 1982). Further studies are needed to clarify these observations; our preliminary findings suggest no abnormalities in event-related potentials.

A negative potential (i.e., the readiness or premovement potential) during the half second or so preceding a willed, voluntary movement has been observed in normal human subjects (Kornhuber and Deecke 1965) and in patients with TS (Obeso et al. 1982) following a request by the investigator to mimic a movement. These premovement potentials were not observed in TS patients preceding tics (Obeso et al. 1982). These results have been interpreted as indicating that simple tics are not generated through normal motor pathways utilized for willed movements. In addition, the absence of any observable potential change in the EEG prior to a tic suggests that tics originate in deep brain structures.

Neuropsychological testing of patients with TS has revealed mixed and sometimes conflicting results. Those patients identified as showing evidence of "organicity" have abnormalities compatible with diffuse, nonlocalized, nonspecific CNS dysfunction. Frequently using the age-appropriate Wechsler intelligence scale and/or a test of visual motor integration (VMI; e.g., the Bender-Gestalt), early case reports and surveys of unmedicated TS patients found average or above-average intelligence and VMI impairments. In the largest survey of 144 patients, a normal distribution of overall intelligence and subtest scores was found, except for a significantly increased coding subtest in the Wechsler Intelligence Scale for Children (Corbett et al. 1969). More recent studies have involved some or all subjects on haloperidol and have frequently found normal intelligence quotient (IQ), VMI delays of

≥2 years, and a significant decrease on coding subtests (Friedhoff and Chase 1982). A number of studies suggest that older patients (who have had their TS symptoms longer) have more impairments.

Neuropathology

Only two detailed neuropathological descriptions of cases of TS have been reported in the literature (Richardson 1982). One study found no evidence of a disease process; the other was interpreted as compatible with hypoplasia of the corpus striatum. Currently, there is insufficient neuropathological evidence to suggest a pathological-anatomical correlate of TS. However, recent studies using positron emission tomography (PET) scanning at Johns Hopkins University have suggested alterations in basal ganglia function.

ANIMAL MODELS

Several animal models, most of which involve the pharmacological induction of stereotypic behavior, are being studied for their relevance to TS (Friedhoff and Chase 1982). Particularly intriguing is a model that involves stimulant-induced stereotypic behavior in the rat that is amplified by stress (Knott and Hutson 1982; Leckman et al. 1984).

ASSESSMENT

The History: Interviews and Assessment Instruments

The assessment of a child with TS usually requires a number of hours spent with the child and family. It is important to determine the onset, progression, waxing and waning, and factors that have worsened or ameliorated the expression of motor and phonic tics. It is useful to monitor symptoms over a few months in order to assess their severity and fluctuation, impact on the family, and the nature of the child's and family's adaptation. This monitoring can be facilitated if the family keeps records or uses standard rating forms (e.g., a list of tic symptoms and a behavioral checklist).

Other areas of functioning, particularly school performance, attentional and learning difficulties, and relationships with family members and peers, require careful evaluation. By the time of the evaluation, the child may be extremely distressed by his or her own experiences and by the criticism he or she may have received from the parents who may have scolded, cajoled, bribed, threatened, and punished in order to get the child to stop this "weird" and embarrassing behavior.

Previous medications need to be reviewed in detail. If a child had received stimulant medications, it is important to determine why the medication was prescribed, whether there were any preexisting tics or compulsions, and the temporal relation between the stimulants and new symptoms. Catecholamine agonists are contained in other drugs, such as in antihistamine combinations used in treating allergies and in medications used for asthma. If such drugs were used in the past, it is important to know their effects. Children who developed tics on stimulants may have shown improved attention and learning with the use of these medications.

Frequently, children will have been tried on other medications before being assessed by the current clinician. The child's response to these medications, the dosages used, the initial positive and negative responses, and the rationale for their discontinuation need to be assessed. A family may report that haloperidol was not useful for a child or that it induced unacceptable side effects. A careful history may reveal that the child improved on haloperidol but then developed akathisia, which was not recognized, or that the side effects were dose related and probably controllable. Was the medication used at the correct dosage, with good monitoring, for a long enough time? Patients and families may not recognize important side effects such as fearfulness or school phobia that may be related to haloperidol and not primarily to psychological issues.

The great variability in symptomatic expression seen in TS patients—the waxing and waning course, the exacerbation pro-

Table 1 Tourette Syndrome Global Scale

Code for Frequency
1 = one or less in 5 min
2 = one in 2–4.9 min
3 = from one in 1.9 min to four in 1 min
4 = five or more in 1 min
5 = virtually uncountable

| | Frequency (F) | | | | | | Disruption (D) | | | | | Subscore |
	None	Rarely	Occasionally	Frequently	Almost Always	Always	Camouflaged	Audible or Visible, No problem	Some problem	Impaired Functioning	Cannot Function	
Simple Motor (SM) Nonpurposeful tics, jerks, and/or movements	0	1	2	3	4	5	1	2	3	4	5	$F \times D =$ ___
Complex Motor (CM) Purposeful, thoughtful actions (systematic actions; rituals; touching self, others, or objects)	0	1	2	3	4	5	1	2	3	4	5	$F \times D =$ ___
Simple Phonic (SP) Nonpurposeful noises, throat clearing, coughing	0	1	2	3	4	5	1	2	3	4	5	$F \times D =$ ___
Complex Phonic (CP) Purposeful; insults; coprolalia; words distinguishable	0	1	2	3	4	5	1	2	3	4	5	$F \times D =$ ___

Behavior (Conduct) (B)

0 No problem
5 Subtle problems; normal peer, school, and family relations
10 Some problems; at least one relationship area impaired
15 Clear impairment in more than one area
20 Serious impairment; affects all areas
25 Unacceptable social behavior; needs constant supervision

Motor Restlessness (MR)

0 Normal movement
5 Adventitious movements; visible; no problem
10 Increased motor restlessness; clearly visible; some problem
15 Clear motor restlessness; moderate problem
20 Mostly in motion but occasionally stops; impaired functioning
25 Nonstop motion; clearly cannot function

School and Learning Problems

0 No problem
5 Low grades
10 Should be (or already in) some special classes, or repeated a grade
15 All special classes
20 Special school
25 Unable to remain in school, homebound

Work and Occupation Problems

0 No problem
5 Stable job, some difficulty
10 Serious problems
15 Lost many jobs
20 Almost never employed
25 Unemployed

$[(SM + CM)/2] + [(SP + CP)/2] + [(B + MR + \text{school or work problems}) + 2/3] = \text{global score} = \underline{\hspace{1cm}}$

NOTE. From Harcherik et al. (1984).

duced by stress or anxiety, and the ability of many TS patients to control their symptoms for brief periods of time—can lead to a bewildering clinical picture that the patient, parents, teacher, and clinician each "see" differently. Information obtained from multiple sources over the longest possible period of time is essential for clarifying the clinical picture so that a consensus can emerge regarding the patient's strengths and problems and the nature of the symptomatic fluctuations. The use of standardized clinical assessment instruments, which are usually developed and employed for research purposes, can help in elucidating many clinical issues. We ask parents to complete a standardized questionnaire that assesses the child's current and past symptoms and development. In addition, parents intermittently fill out a checklist that measures symptom severity. Teachers are also intermittently asked to complete a symptom checklist. We currently use the Tourette Syndrome Global Scale (see Table 1) for our clinical ratings. Various assessment instruments for TS currently are being evaluated for validity and reliability by our group, as well as by others.

As the evaluation proceeds and the child becomes more comfortable, he or she will reveal symptoms with less suppression or inhibition. Only when there is confidence in the doctor is a child or adult likely to acknowledge the most frightening and bizarre symptoms (e.g., "disgusting" habits, obsessive thoughts, or rituals). A well-conducted assessment allows the family to feel that their full story has been heard—sometimes for the first time after having seen many physicians. This assessment process can be therapeutically important and lead to an easing of the immediate crisis. In addition, nothing is more useful for developing confidence than the family's and child's belief that the clinician has "heard" what they have been through and understands how they are coping with the tragedy they have experienced.

Behavioral Pedigree of the Extended Family

It is of interest to have a detailed behavioral pedigree of the extended family, including tics, attentional problems, learning disorders, and compulsions. A grandfather's TS may have been diagnosed as Sydenham's chorea; an uncle may have been thought simply to be odd or weird. Parents may be embarrassed about acknowledging their own symptoms—if a father is asked about his obvious eye-blinking and throat-clearing tics, he may initially deny that he has ever had tics or that he ever noticed them. Only when the mother comments on noticing them "when he's nervous" will he be able to "remember" his childhood and current symptoms.

Cognitive Function

Careful assessment of cognitive functioning and school achievement is indicated for children having school problems. The nature of this assessment can be similar to that for other children with school performance problems. TS children with cognitive difficulties rarely have clearly delineated learning disorders, and the average IQ of TS patients is normal; rather, their problems include distractibility, perseveration, and difficulty in keeping themselves and their work organized. Many have difficulties with penmanship (graphomotor skills) and compulsions that interfere with writing. Determining specific problem areas will help in the recommendation of alternatives (e.g., the use of a typewriter or more emphasis on oral reports).

Neurological Examination

Neurological examination should include documentation of neuromaturational difficulties as well as other neurological findings. About half of TS patients have nonlocalizing, so-called "soft" neurological findings suggesting disturbances in the body schema and integration of motor control. Although these findings have no specific therapeutic implications, they probably strengthen the diagnosis of TS and may define a clinical subgroup. Neurological observations also are important as "baseline" data since the use of medications may cloud the neurological picture.

Children with paroxysmally abnormal EEG tracings sometimes

have been treated as epileptic, but anticonvulsants are of no consistent value in TS. CT of the brain generally produces normal results, and the EEG and CT are not necessary for the diagnosis or treatment of TS. Yet, concerned clinicians are likely to feel comforted by a normal EEG and CT scan; at the least, certain other disorders affecting movement (such as seizures or basal ganglia disorders) are more or less ruled out.

Laboratory Tests

No diagnostic laboratory tests are specific for TS. Chemical studies may include electrolytes, calcium, phosphorus, ceruloplasmin, and liver function tests—all related to movement difficulties of various types.

Assessment Problems

Although prevailing diagnostic criteria would require that all children with suppressible multiple motor and phonic tics, however minimal, for at least 1 year be diagnosed as having TS, in practice we deviate from this rigorous research approach. In talking with families, we tend to consider severity and associated features (particularly complex motor and phonic symptoms, as well as attention problems and general disinhibition) in the diagnosis of TS. For the meticulous, hard-working boy, we are willing to use the term "nervous habits" to cover his throat clearing, facial grimacing, and occasional shrugging. However, since there are genetic implications, and some families and patients will want to have full disclosure of the physician's thoughts, the clinician may want to raise the possible relationship between the patient's symptoms and TS. The problem is that, whereas not everyone who twitches has TS, in the absence of diagnostic tests it may be hard to draw the line. For research purposes, it is necessary to maintain clear diagnostic criteria.

When a child is currently on a medication but is still having serious tic or behavioral difficulties, hard clinical judgment is called for. Today, TS patients will frequently be on haloperidol, clonidine, a phenothiazine, or some combination of drugs at the time of evaluation. The clinician will have to decide whether to increase the medication(s) and see if the child improves or discontinue the medication(s) and observe the child's response. Discontinuation of haloperidol may lead to severe withdrawal-emergent exacerbation for up to 2–3 months. Thus, if haloperidol is withdrawn, it cannot be expected that the child's "real" status will be visible for quite a while. Some children may improve for a few weeks after haloperidol discontinuation and then exacerbate after another week or so, remain worse for a while, and gradually improve. With discontinuation of haloperidol, cognitive blunting, feeling dull, decreased motivation, social phobias, excessive appetite, and sedation may lift rather quickly, over days to several weeks, while emergent tic symptoms remain or become worse. Thus, the decision to discontinue haloperidol must be planned so as to disrupt the child's life as little as possible.

If a child is on clonidine and is not benefiting, tapering the medication over 1 or 2 weeks may be followed by a brief period of exacerbation lasting from several days to a few weeks. This exacerbation typically is milder than that with haloperidol withdrawal. Infrequently, children seem to get worse during withdrawal than they were before the initiation of treatment. Less is known about withdrawal from phenothiazines, but withdrawal-emergent dyskinesias and exacerbations can occur.

A clinician will have to decide whether to attempt to "clean out" a child's system by discontinuation of all medication or to change dosage when symptoms are poorly controlled. The presence of serious side effects would probably lead us to attempt detoxification, but careful assessment of the child's and family's coping and response to intervention can guide such decisions.

Another complication encountered during the assessment of a child with TS is that the parents themselves may have TS or an associated disorder. There are several implications of this multigenerational sharing of symptoms. Clinicians may feel inhibited in fully sharing their impressions of the child's social and personality problems if they observe similar difficulties in the parents, for fear that they may hurt their feelings. Also, parents may feel an additional burden of guilt if they recognize that they have contributed genetically to their child's disorder. On the other side, parents with TS or tics may have more sympathy for their child's dilemmas and greater capacity to appreciate how life can proceed in spite of them. In addition, they may be interested in receiving treatment for themselves, or other family members, if there is success in the treatment of the child.

Families frequently ask if TS is a "medical" or "emotional" disorder. These terms carry with them ideological and psychological weight. A well-conducted assessment, in which all aspects of the child's development and current functioning are discussed, is an important step in undoing an epistemologically mischievous disjunction between an isolated body and a detached mind. Whereas it is clear that TS arises on the basis of neurophysiological dysfunction, and thus is "biological," it is equally apparent that its manifestations affect the child in many areas of his or her life. Thus, the treatment of TS must address the child as a whole person and not just as a collection of physical symptoms. This orientation to TS and its treatment can be conveyed implicitly during the assessment—as the clinician analyzes medical, psychosocial, and psychological issues—and usually requires explicit discussion at the end of the evaluation.

MANAGEMENT

Effective treatment is now available for many patients with TS. There are several approaches to therapy.

Monitoring

Initially, unless there is a state of emergency, the clinician can follow the patient for several months before deciding with the family on a specific treatment plan (Cohen et al. 1984). The goals of this first stage of treatment are to establish a baseline of symptoms; define associated difficulties in school, family, and peer relations; obtain necessary medical tests; monitor, through checklists and interviews, the range of and fluctuations in symptoms and the specific areas of greatest difficulty; and establish a relationship. If there is an ongoing exposure to stimulants, they should be discontinued if medically feasible.

Education and Reassurance

Families vary in their understanding of TS and their ideas about prognosis. In addition to their personal experience, what patients and parents have read or been told may greatly influence their perception of the syndrome. Patients and families deserve a frank discussion of available treatments, prognosis, and emerging knowledge of genetic factors. Given the availability of effective treatments, we are generally optimistic when discussing prognosis. Literature from the Tourette Syndrome Association (41-02 Bell Blvd., Bayside, NY 11361) and professional journals may also be helpful.

Medication

Available pharmacological agents are effective in suppressing the symptoms of TS in the majority of patients. However, drugs are not curative, and patients may need to continue them for extended periods of time.

Haloperidol. Since the early 1960s, haloperidol (Haldol) has been the drug of choice in treating TS. This agent has been found effective in numerous clinical studies, and its use for the control of TS symptoms has been approved by the Food and Drug Administration (FDA) (Shapiro and Shapiro 1982). Haloperidol is most effective at low doses. It is not unusual for patients to experience improvement in their symptoms with as little as 0.5 mg/day p.o. Haloperidol's effectiveness in controlling symptoms can usually be determined after several days at a given dosage level. The dose is usually not to be increased more rapidly than 0.5 mg every 3–7 days. At doses of >1 mg/day, a divided dosage regimen is usually best. The higher the dose, the more likely are unwanted physical and psychological effects. Patients, of whatever age, rarely have a favorable response to >5 mg/day. Even if the medication has been effective in controlling the tics, its side effects are judged by many patients and their families to be worse than the disorder. Indeed, only about 30 percent of patients who have had a favorable response choose to remain on this medication long term (>1 year). Although some patients, particularly those on low doses, do not experience any side effects on haloperidol, many do. These include dysphoria, depression, phobias, sedation, cognitive dulling, excessive weight gain, acute dystonic reaction, parkinsonian symptoms, and akathisia. The extrapyramidal side effects may be effectively treated with antiparkinsonian medications such as benztropine (Cogentin). Prolonged use of haloperidol carries a risk of inducing tardive dyskinesia.

Clonidine. The first report in 1979 of the value of clonidine (Catapres) in treating TS has been followed by other case reports and open and blind trials suggesting that from 40 to 70 percent of TS patients benefit from its use (Cohen et al. 1980; Leckman et al. 1982). Clonidine has been approved by the FDA only for use in hypertension, but clinicians can prescribe it without special government approval for TS as long as they understand its indications and share the basis for their decision with the family and child. Formal FDA approval of the drug's use in TS is likely. Many groups are currently using clonidine as the first drug because of its relative safety and the low occurrence of side effects. Although many patients with TS have a favorable response to clonidine, this favorable outcome often takes 2–3 months to develop. The reasons for this latency of response are not clear. In general, clonidine is started at low doses of 0.05 mg/day, and slowly titrated over several weeks to 0.15–0.30 mg/day. Doses of >0.5 mg/day may be beneficial, but often lead to undesirable side effects. As with haloperidol, the best responses are in those patients who respond at the lower dosages. At low doses, the side effects of clonidine include fatigue that usually "wears off" after several weeks, and dry mouth. At higher doses, orthostatic hypotension can occur. Prolongation of the PR interval has been reported. Untoward psychological effects, including increased irritability, have also been reported at higher doses. In addition to the usual workup described above, a baseline electrocardiogram (ECG) should be obtained prior to the initiation of clonidine.

Pimozide. Pimozide (Orap) is a potent neuroleptic widely used in Europe in the treatment of psychosis; several open and blind clinical studies have shown it to be at least as effective as haloperidol in the treatment of TS (Ross and Moldolfsky 1977; Shapiro et al. 1983; Shapiro and Shapiro 1984). Pimozide is a diphenylbutylpiperidine derivative, chemically distinct from haloperidol, clonidine, or the phenothiazines. Its mode of action appears to be a preferential inhibition of postsynaptic DA receptors.

Treatment with pimozide is initiated at 1 mg/day, and dosage is gradually increased, on clinical indications, to a maximum of 6–10 mg/day (0.2 mg/kg) for children and 20 mg/day for adults. Pimozide's long half-life (55 hr) makes once-daily dosage possible. Major side effects are similar to those described for haloperidol. Pimozide also causes ECG changes in up to 25 percent of patients, including T-wave inversion, U waves, QT prolongation, and bradycardia. Such changes are observable within 1 week and at doses as low as 3 mg/day. The manufacturer recommends discontinuation of pimozide with the occurrence of T-wave inversion or U waves, seen in up to 20 percent of patients; dosage should not be increased if there is a prolongation of the QT interval (corrected). At least three cardiac deaths have occurred in healthy young men. As with haloperidol, tardive dyskinesia must be considered a long-term possibility. In addition to the usual clinical and laboratory monitoring, patients receiving pimozide should receive regular ECG monitoring.

Other Medications. A variety of other medications, particularly neuroleptics, have been used to treat patients with TS (Friedhoff and Chase 1982). Some phenothiazines may be as effective as haloperidol. Agents that affect primarily serotonergic or cholinergic systems, although interesting from a research perspective, have not found a place in the treatment of TS.

Choice of Medication. The clinician's choice of a first drug is a difficult decision. Haloperidol has the longest "track record," and its therapeutic benefits and side effects are well defined. The only other major contender as a first drug today is clonidine, the action of which is less well defined and which is less likely to be dramatically effective. Those clinicians who favor clonidine as a first drug do so because of its limited side effects and positive effect on attention; however, where a rapid response is needed, haloperidol may be more effective. Until more evidence accumulates, it will be difficult to decide if a patient should have a several-month course of clonidine before starting haloperidol or the other way round. If a patient is started on haloperidol, it may be more difficult to discontinue because of withdrawal symptoms, which are usually less severe with clonidine at usual doses. Some clinicians have added low-dose clonidine to low-dose haloperidol with good results, but no controlled studies have yet been reported. Whether pimozide will become an alternative to haloperidol may depend on the seriousness and frequency of its side effects.

Academic Intervention

Children with attentional and learning problems require educational intervention similar to the approaches used in the management of other forms of ADD and learning disabilities. TS patients may require special tutoring, a learning laboratory, a self-contained classroom, a special school, or residential school, depending on the severity of school-related and other behavioral problems. It may be difficult to convince a school district of the need for special school provisions for a bright TS patient who does not have specific learning disabilities but whose attentional problems limit his or her optimal functioning. Since TS is an uncommon disorder, schools need to be informed about the nature of TS and the ways it affects attention and learning. A homebound program, which deprives children of their legal right to the least restrictive educational environment and an adequate education, should be avoided.

Genetic Counseling

Parents and older TS patients want to know about the genetic risk for siblings and offspring. Since the precise mode of inheritance is still not known, only generalizations are possible. Parents considering having another child should be told that having a first-degree relative (parent or sibling) with TS increases the risk of having the disorder from one in many hundreds or thousands to one in four or five. The risk is much higher for male offspring. For a young adult with TS who is thinking about having a child, genetic counseling must be done cautiously and with sensitivity regarding the meaning of the information. As previously noted, the offspring of a mother with TS are at quite a high risk. At present, there is no method for prenatal diagnosis. In providing genetic counseling, it is important to emphasize the uncertainties, as well as the increasing knowledge, about treatment.

Psychotherapy and Rehabilitation

Psychotherapy is probably not effective in reducing tics. However, psychotherapy and other counseling techniques can help patients and their families adjust more easily to life with TS.

Short-term hospitalization may be useful during crises. Because phonic symptoms and bizarre behaviors may be difficult to tolerate in the hospital, TS patients are often unwelcome on an inpatient neurology or psychiatry service. When patients are hospitalized, there is a tendency to use medication for sedation, not only because of the patient's needs, but because of the anxiety of the clinical staff and other patients. Yet, the availability of an inpatient service willing to accept a TS patient in crisis can be reassuring for both the patient and the physician.

For the young adult who has had serious difficulties with school achievement, socialization, and personality development, a thorough rehabilitation program is required. The patient may need vocational guidance, a halfway house program, psychotherapy, family counseling, and advocacy, in addition to judicious use of medication. Even in desperate situations, therapeutic commitment combined with the patient's determination and courage may lead to satisfying therapeutic results.

FUTURE DEVELOPMENTS

Basic and clinical researchers are currently attempting to elucidate the etiology, pathogenesis, and most effective treatment of TS. Recent developments in human behavioral genetics may soon be joined by those in molecular biology and result in the identification of the genetic defect(s) underlying the disorder. New imaging techniques such as nuclear magnetic resonance and PET will allow for greater understanding of the anatomical structures and metabolic processes involved in the pathogenesis of TS. The use of medication challenges may add another dimension to our understanding of neurochemistry (Leckman et al 1982). In addition, as our basic and clinical knowledge of TS increases, we can expect new medications to be developed that will more specifically treat the underlying defect(s) in this syndrome.

References

American Psychiatric Association: Diagnostic and Statistical Manual of Mental Disorders, 3rd ed. Washington, DC, American Psychiatric Association, 1980

Antelman SM, Caggiula AR: Norepinephrine-dopamine interactions and behavior. Science 195:646–653, 1977

Bergen D, Tanner CM, Wilson R: The electroencephalogram in Tourette syndrome. Ann Neurol 11:382–385, 1982

Bliss J, Cohen DJ, Freedman DX: Sensory experiences of Gilles de la Tourette syndrome. Arch Gen Psychiatry 37:1343–1347, 1980

Borison RL, Ang L, Chang S, et al: New pharmacological approaches in the treatment of Gilles de la Tourette syndrome, in Advances in

Neurology, Vol 35: Gilles de la Tourette Syndrome. Edited by Freid-hoff AJ, Chase TN. New York, Raven Press, 1982, pp 377–382

Bunney BS, DeRiemer SA: Effects of clonidine on nigral dopamine cell activity: possible mediation by noradrenergic regulation of seroton-ergic raphe system, in Advances in Neurology, Vol 35: Gilles de la Tourette Syndrome. Edited by Friedhoff AJ, Chase TN. New York, Raven Press, 1982, pp 99–104

Butler IJ, Koslow S, Seifert W, et al: Biogenic amine metabolism in Tourette syndrome. Ann Neurol 6:37–39, 1979

Caparulo BK, Cohen DJ, Rothman SL, et al: Computed tomographic brain scanning in children with developmental neuropsychiatric disorders. J Am Acad Child Psychiatry 20:338–357, 1981

Cohen DJ, Shaywitz BA, Young JG, et al: Central biogenic amine metabolism in children with the syndrome of chronic multiple tics of Gilles de la Tourette syndrome: norepinephrine, serotonin, and dopa-mine. J Am Acad Child Psychiatry 18:320–341, 1979

Cohen DJ, Detlor J, Young JG, et al: Clonidine ameliorates Gilles de la Tourette syndrome. Arch Gen Psychiatry 37:1350–1357, 1980

Cohen DJ, Detlor J, Shaywitz BA, et al: Interaction of biological and psychological factors in the natural history of Tourette's syndrome: a paradigm for childhood neuropsychiatric disorders, in Advances in Neurology, Vol 35: Gilles de la Tourette Syndrome. Edited by Fried-hoff AJ, Chase TN. New York, Raven Press, 1982, pp 31–40

Cohen DJ, Leckman JF, Shaywitz BA: Tourette's syndrome: assessment and treatment, in Diagnosis and Treatment in Pediatric Psychiatry. Edited by Shaffer D, Ehrhardt AA, Greenhill L. New York, Macmillan (in press)

Corbett JA, Matthews AM, Connell PH, et al: Tics and Gilles de la Tourette syndrome: a follow-up study and critical review. Br J Psychia-try 115:1229–1241, 1969

Domino EF, Piggott L, Demetriou S, et al: Visually evoked responses in

Tourette syndrome, in Advances in Neurology, Vol 35: Gilles de la Tourette Syndrome. Edited by Friedhoff AJ, Chase TN. New York, Raven Press, 1982, pp 115–120

Feinberg M, Carroll BJ: Effects of dopamine agonists and antagonists in Tourette's disease. Arch Gen Psychiatry 36:979–985, 1979

Friedhoff AJ: Receptor maturation in pathogenesis and treatment of Tourette syndrome, in Advances in Neurology, Vol 35: Gilles de la Tourette Syndrome. Edited by Friedhoff AJ, Chase TN. New York, Raven Press, 1982, pp 133–140

Friedhoff AJ, Chase TN, eds: Advances in Neurology, Vol 35: Gilles de la Tourette Syndrome. New York, Raven Press, 1982

Gilles de la Tourette G: Etude sur une affection nerveuse, caracterisée par de l'incoordination motrice, acompagnée d'echolalie et de coprolalia. Arch Neurol (Paris) 9:19–42, 1885

Goetz CG, Klawans HL: Gilles de la Tourette on Tourette syndrome, in Advances in Neurology, Vol 35: Gilles de la Tourette Syndrome. Edited by Friedhoff AJ, Chase TN. New York, Raven Press, 1982, pp 1–16

Golden GS: Gilles de la Tourette's syndrome following methylphenidate administration. Dev Med Child Neurol 16:76–78, 1974

Hanin I, Merikangas JR, Merikangas KR, et al: Red-cell choline and Gilles de la Tourette syndrome. N Engl J Med 301:661–662, 1979

Harcherik DF, Leckman JF, Detlor J: A new instrument for clinical studies of Tourette syndrome. J Am Acad Child Psychiatry 23:153–160, 1984

Hoder EL, Leckman JF, Ehrenkranz R, et al: Clonidine in neonatal narcotic abstinence syndrome. N Engl J Med 305:1284, 1981

Jagger J, Prusoff BA, Cohen DJ, et al: The epidemiology of Tourette's syndrome: a pilot study. Schizophr Bull 8:267–278, 1982

Knott PJ, Hutson PH: Stress-induced stereotypy in the rat: neuropharmacological similarities to Tourette syndrome, in Advances in Neurology, Vol 35: Gilles de la Tourette Syndrome. Edited by Friedhoff AJ, Chase TN. New York, Raven Press, 1982, pp 233–238

Kornhuber HH, Deecke L: Hirnpotentialanderungen bei Willkurbewegungen und passiven Bewegungen des Menschen: Bereitschaftspotential und reafferente Potentiale. Pflugers Arch 284:1–17, 1965

Leckman JF, Maas JW, Redmond DE Jr, et al: Effects of oral clonidine on plasma 3-methoxy-4-hydroxyphenethylene glycol (MHPG) in man: preliminary report. Life Sci 26:2179–2185, 1980

Leckman JF, Maas JW, Heninger GR: Covariance of plasma free 3-methoxy-4-hydroxyphenethylene glycol and diastolic blood pressure. Eur J Pharmacol 70:111–120, 1981

Leckman JF, Cohen DJ, Detlor J, et al: Clonidine in the treatment of Gilles de la Tourette syndrome: a review, in Advances in Neurology, Vol 35: Gilles de la Tourette Syndrome. Edited by Friedhoff AJ, Chase TN. New York, Raven Press, 1982, pp 391–402

Leckman JF, Detlor J, Harcherik DF, et al: Acute and chronic clonidine treatment in Tourette's syndrome: a preliminary report on clinical response and effect on plasma and urinary catecholamine metabolites, growth hormone, and blood pressure. J Am Acad Child Psychiatry 22:433–440, 1983

Leckman JF, Cohen DJ, Price RA, et al: The pathogenesis of Gilles de la Tourette syndrome: a review of data and hypotheses, in Movement Disorders. Edited by Shah NS, Donald A. New York, Plenum Press (in press)

Lowe TL, Cohen DJ, Detlor J, et al: Stimulant medications precipitate Tourette's syndrome. JAMA 247:1729–1731, 1982

Obesco JA, Rothwell JC, Marsden CD: The Neurophysiology of Tourette syndrome, in Advances in Neurology, Vol 35: Gilles de la Tourette Syndrome. Edited by Friedhoff AJ, Chase TN. New York, Raven Press, 1982, pp 105–114

Pauls DL, Cohen DJ, Heimbuch R, et al: Familial patterns and transmission of Gilles de la Tourette syndrome and multiple tics. Arch Gen Psychiatry 38:1085–1090, 1981

Pauls DL, Kruger SD, Leckman JF, et al: The risk of Tourette syndrome (TS) and chronic multiple tics (CMT) among relatives of TS patients obtained by direct interview. J Am Acad Child Psychiatry 23:134–137, 1984

Richardson EP Jr: Neuropathological studies of Tourette syndrome, in Advances in Neurology, Vol 35: Gilles de la Tourette Syndrome. Edited by Friedhoff AJ, Chase TN. New York, Raven Press, 1982, pp 83–87

Ross MS, Moldofsky H: Comparison of pimozide with haloperidol in Gilles de la Tourette syndrome. Lancet 1:103, 1977

Shapiro AK, Shapiro E: Clinical efficacy of haloperidol, pimozide, penfluridol, and clonidine in the treatment of Tourette syndrome, in Advances in Neurology, Vol 35: Gilles de la Tourette Syndrome. Edited by Friedhoff AJ, Chase TN. New York, Raven Press, 1982, pp 383–386

Shapiro AK, Shapiro E: Controlled study of pimozide vs placebo in Tourette syndrome. J Am Acad Child Psychiatry 23:161–173, 1984

Shapiro AK, Shapiro E, Bruun RD, et al: Gilles de la Tourette syndrome. New York, Raven Press, 1978

Shapiro AK, Shapiro E, Eisenkraft GJ: Treatment of Gilles de la Tourette syndrome with pimozide. Am J Psychiatry 140:1183–1186, 1983

Stahl SM, Berger PA: Cholinergic and dopaminergic mechanisms in Tourette syndrome, in Advances in Neurology, Vol 35: Gilles de la Tourette Syndrome. Edited by Friedhoff AJ, Chase TN. New York, Raven Press, 1982, pp 141–150

Volkmar FR, Leckman JF, Cohen DJ, et al: EEG abnormalities in Tourette's syndrome. J Am Acad Child Psychiatry 23:32–353, 1984

3

Huntington's Disease

Nancy Wexler, Ph.D.

3

Huntington's Disease

At the close of the tenure of the Congressional Commission for the Control of Huntington's Disease and Its Consequences in 1977, for which I served as Executive Director, copies of the final report were sent to departments of neurology and psychiatry around the country. One psychiatry department chairperson at a prestigious school wrote back an irate letter scolding us for wasting taxpayers' money by sending him the report since everybody knows that Huntington's disease (HD) is not a psychiatric disorder. I am doubly pleased at the inclusion of a chapter on HD in this monograph, suggesting that psychiatrists believe that this fascinating and mysterious illness is within their purview of interest.

George Huntington certainly did not think that this disorder that bears his name had no relevance for psychiatry. In addition to being the first to accurately describe its Mendelian inheritance pattern, years before Mendel's laws were rediscovered, he insightfully depicted HD as "that insanity tending towards suicide" (Huntington 1872).

HD is an autosomal, dominantly inherited disorder that affects almost all aspects of mental and physical functioning: movement, mood, and mental ability. The HD gene is located on chromosome 4 (Gusella et al. 1983).

EPIDEMIOLOGY

HD was once thought to be extremely rare, but is now considered to be among the more common autosomal dominant disorders. Prevalence rates, or the numbers of cases ascertained in a given time and place, have varied between 5 and 10 per 100,000 individuals in the population. The prevalence rate for blacks appears to be one-third the rate for whites, and Orientals have only one-tenth the prevalence (Conneally 1984). These racial differences may be spurious owing to ascertainment and diagnostic errors or they may serve as evidence for one hypothesis, espoused by Kurtzke (1979), that the HD mutation is an ancient one occurring in western Europe and brought to Africa and the Orient through trade and migration. Certainly, the mutation rate for HD is among the lowest known for human disorders (from 1.3×10^{7} to 5.4×10^{-6}) (Conneally 1984). In fact, no new mutation has ever been documented, although there are some potential candidates now being investigated.

Data on 169 cases with onset before 1960 from the National Institute of Neurological and Communicative Disorders and Stroke National Huntington's Disease Research Roster at Indiana University indicate that there has been no change over time in the duration of the disease, despite some palliative treatments and probably somewhat better care. Perhaps more notable is the rise in the number of cases during the first part of the twentieth century, probably owing to population growth, increased physician awareness, and improved diagnosis (Conneally 1984).

GENETICS

The impressive array of psychological and motoric symptomatology of HD results from a single gene defect (as far as we know), with delayed onset and complete penetrance. Each child of a parent with the illness has a 50 percent risk of inheriting it. Onset is usually in the third or forth decade. Although there is currently no test that can detect the presence of the gene before symptoms of the disease appear, a linkage test using a newly discovered DNA marker that can indicate the presence or absence of the gene is now under development and should be available as soon as it can be determined that there is no genetic heterogeneity, that is, more than one HD gene. The HD gene carrier will eventually develop the disease, if he or she lives long enough; in this sense, the illness does not "skip generations"; i.e., it does not remain quiescent in one generation to reappear in the next. If a child does not inherit the gene, transmission is impossible and the disease disappears from that line.

The juvenile form of HD is an intriguing puzzle. Approximately three-fourths of the affected children under the age of 20, both male and female, inherit the disease from their father. As the age at onset becomes younger, the likelihood that the father transmits the gene approaches 100 percent. No one knows what causes this deviation from Mendelian expectations (Boehnke et al. 1983).

There are few forces that conspire to take this late-onset disorder out of the gene pool, other than voluntary abstinence from childbearing. A community in Venezuela demonstrates what happens when the gene flourishes unchecked. We have been able to trace this particular gene back to some time in the early 1800s to a woman living in a village built on stilts over the water. From her, there is now a population of 3,500 descendants and their families living along the shores of Lake Maracaibo, Venezuela. All the HD patients in this population have inherited the same HD gene from this common ancestor, thus providing a huge research population with genetic homogeneity for the illness. Currently there are about 88 living HD patients and 1,528 persons at 50 or 25 percent risk.

CLINICAL PICTURE

HD is characterized by an array of involuntary and abnormal movements in all parts of the body, cognitive decline, and affective disorders or symptomatology resembling schizophrenia. The most frequent misdiagnoses given to HD patients are Parkinson's disease and schizophrenia, although tardive dyskinesia, Alhzeimer's disease, and multiple sclerosis are also common. Until deinstitutionalization policies changed psychiatric hospital clientele, institutionalized HD patients were usually found in state psychiatric hospitals. Now the majority are cared for at home or in nursing homes.

The variable age at onset has a major impact on the psychology of HD. The majority of cases have onset between the ages of 30 and 50, but the range is very wide. Although the odds decline after the age of 40, individuals at risk know that there is still some chance of developing the illness as late as the eighth decade (Conneally 1984). Couples worry not only that the spouse at risk may become ill, but also that their children will develop the disorder. Since the majority of juvenile cases come from affected fathers and often aggregate within families, it is not uncommon to find families in which a mother has just buried a spouse and has one or two or even as many as four affected children at home. The dominant transmission, delayed age at onset, and long duration of the illness mean that two generations are often affected at the same time, or that offspring have just finished nursing a parent through the rather ghastly terminal phases of the illness when their own diagnosis is made.

There is a rather wide range in the duration of the disease, from 10 to 20 years, with some tendency for the duration to increase as the age at onset becomes older. [In old age, duration may be limited by a shortened life span owing to other causes (Conneally 1984).] The progressive decline in HD is inexorable.

Age at onset data and duration statistics have a wide margin of error because of the insidiousness of the initial symptoms of HD. Age at diagnosis can be 5–10 years after onset.

Although chorea, or semipurposeless, nonstereotyped, involuntary movement, is the predominant motor abnormality in HD, other motor disorders can coexist. Dystonia and parkinsonian symptoms begin somewhat later in the illness and progressively worsen. Some patients have a variant (Westphal variant) that is rigid and parkinsonian from the start, including tremor and bradykinesia. The juvenile cases are almost all rigid, and many have seizures. There is usually a mixed picture, in juveniles as well as adults, of chorea, rigidity, parkinsonism, and dystonia. Muscle tone can be either increased or decreased, and motor impersistence is characteristic. Oculomotor abnormalities are early changes in the illness, often giving the patient a kind of "gluey" or stupid look before other signs are noticeable. Optokinetic nystagmus is lost, and vertical and horizontal smooth pursuit is impaired. Patients are unable to track a stimulus without interrupting their gaze and are unable to move their eyes without moving their heads.

Accurate information on causes of death is difficult to obtain, but aspiration pneumonia and heart disease are common. In the Roster data, suicide and choking were equally frequent causes of death, each accounting for approximately 5 percent of 241 HD deaths (Conneally 1984). The end stage is characterized by severe cachexia, incontinence, dysarthria beyond comprehension, and the inability to eat, walk, or perform any activity independently.

PSYCHIATRIC ASPECTS

Dramatic as the abnormal movements are in HD, most patients and families complain of the psychiatric problems as being the most distressing. These difficulties seem to be a combination of endogenous and reactive symptoms, making them difficult for the physician, as well as the patient and family, to disentangle. The most common psychiatric disorders are depression, usually unipolar but occasionally bipolar, episodic dyscontrol syndromes as defined by Diagnostic and Statistical Manual of Mental Disorders (3rd edition; DSM-III) criteria (American Psychiatric Association 1980), irritability, and apathy (see Chapter 6). Patients may have rage attacks, sometimes lasting hours or days, and may fling furniture about or become violent to others. Often these rampaging periods are triggered by some frustration, such as the inability to be understood or to do something once easily managed. The provocation is often reasonable, while the dyscontrol expressed in the intensity of the reaction is due to the illness.

Understanding the depression associated with HD is complex. Many people assume that depression is certainly a natural, if not appropriate, response to a difficult, stressful, and frightening situation. Yet, it is also an integral part of the disease symptom picture and is variably responsive to tricyclic and other antidepressant therapy.

In a family study stemming from an epidemiological survey of HD in the state of Maryland, Folstein and colleagues (Folstein and Folstein 1983; Folstein et al. 1983) found that 41 percent of HD patients suffered at some time from a major affective disorder. These investigators modified DSM-III criteria (American Psychiatric Association 1980) used to diagnose major affective disorders in the general population by making them even more stringent, requiring a 1-month duration of symptoms instead of 2 weeks. Twenty-eight of the patients had only depressive episodes, whereas eight fluctuated between mania and depression.

The Folstein group then examined family members with HD, ascertained through probands both with and without a major affective disorder. Twenty of the 23 secondary cases also had both HD and manic depressive illness when the proband had both disorders, whereas this characterized only 5 of the 23 secondary cases ascertained through a proband with HD alone. Those with both disorders often have a long history of affective disease as many as 20 years prior to the onset of classic HD symptoms. These data suggest that in families in which affective disorder is a prominent symptom of HD, the illness seems to segregate with the HD gene.

In the Folstein survey, only 2 of the 88 patients ascertained met DSM-III criteria (American Psychiatric Association 1980) for schizophrenia. Although some HD patients have auditory hallucinations or delusions, usually paranoid, these symptoms are not typical of most cases. Often patients are misdiagnosed as schizophrenic because they are unkempt, aggressive, or suspicious. Many patients are now routinely treated with haloperidol (Haldol; although the wisdom of this therapy is questionable) so that the drug may obscure the natural psychiatric picture. In Venezuela, where medications are not used, only 1 of 60 patients examined had visual hallucinations and delusions, while depression was much more common.

Of course, it is also possible to have a psychiatric disorder independent of HD. The appearance of a psychiatric disease in a person at risk cannot be diagnostic of the illness, only suggestive. Even if HD develops eventually, we cannot be certain that a major affective disorder or psychosis 5–10 years before a definitive HD diagnosis is a part of the disease.

Psychiatrists treating at-risk individuals find themselves in the same quandary as their patients. If the patient is depressed or irritable, cannot remember a telephone number, organize a dinner party, or write a paper, bumps into walls on occasion, drops a dish—is it the gene or the reaction? What is the cause? Who in a general psychiatric practice might not qualify for a possible diagnosis of early HD?

Cognitive decline can also precede motoric signs by many years, although usually not as far in advance as emotional disturbances. The intellectual difficulties of HD patients are quite different from the problems of those with Alzheimer's disease or other related dementias. HD patients have trouble with sequential organization, arithmetic, mental manipulation of constructs or images, sustained attention, and memory, particularly short term. Word fluency declines, judgment can be impaired, and the ability to learn new material rapidly and shift set is lost. On the other hand, HD patients generally are oriented to time and place, can recover words with cuing, know their family and friends, have reasonably good insight into their disease, and preserve a sense of humor and "social intelligence." They do not have apraxias, agnosias, or aphasias, and they can understand speech long after their own is unintelligible (Wexler 1979).

NEUROPATHOLOGY

Neuropathologically, the basal ganglia bear the brunt of cell degeneration in HD. Beginning with the dorsal portion of the caudate nucleus and extending throughout the caudate to the putamen, small, spiny, type-II neurons, in particular, die, leaving heavy gliosis and lipofuscin accumulation in their wake. Cell death is also found to a lesser extent in other basal ganglia nuclei, in the third, fifth, and sixth cortical layers, in limbic structures, cerebellum, brainstem, and spinal cord. Not surprisingly with such cell death, neurochemical alterations are also profound (Spokes 1980). Basal ganglia concentrations of γ-aminobutyric acid, acetylcholine, substance P, Met-enkephalin, angiotensin converting enzyme, and cholecystokinin are all reduced. Somatostatin levels are inexplicably elevated, while dopaminergic and glutamatergic pathways are relatively preserved

The work of Kuhl et al. (1982) at the University of California at Los Angeles using positron emission tomography to study glucose metabolism in HD patients and at-risk individuals has demonstrated marked metabolic abnormalities in all of the former and in some of the latter. Their research suggests that when cell death accumulates beyond a certain threshold, compensatory mechanisms do not suffice and symptoms appear.

NEW RESEARCH

Recent advances in molecular genetics hold the best possible prospects for breakthroughs in HD research in both identifying the abnormal gene and developing new treatments. Invetigators at Harvard and other universities began in 1980 to analyze DNA from HD families, looking for a restriction fragment-length polymorphism (RFLP) or structural variation that would indicate the presence of the HD gene. Specific enzymes, called "restriction endonucleases," recognize particular sites in the DNA; when they see such a site, they cut the DNA into fragments. People have different numbers and distributions of these sites, resulting in varying fragment lengths. Patterns of sites and fragment lengths are inherited like genes. There are sufficient numbers of these variations scattered throughout the human genome for one to be sitting fairly close to every gene of interest. The variations become "markers" or "landmarks" in the map of the human genome.

Recently, our team of collaborators (Gusella et al. 1983) succeeded in identifying a polymorphic DNA marker linked to the HD gene. We studied two HD families: a U.S. family of reasonable size and a substantially larger family from Venezuela. In both families, all HD patients and those at risk, particularly individuals older than age 55 and still healthy, were examined neurologically. Blood samples from appropriate individuals were collected. Lymphocytes were separated and transformed with Epstein-Barr virus, and DNS was extracted. Fractions of all blood samples were analyzed for conventional red cell and protein markers to eliminate the rare cases of nonpaternity. On the 13th DNA probe studied, Gusella et al. discovered an RFLP linked within 10 cM to the gene in the two families. The marker, called G8, was localized to chromosome 4 (Gusella et al. 1983). There are four haplotypes of the marker, making it excellent for analysis. The heterogeneity rate in the general population is 57 percent. The next crucial steps will be to isolate the HD gene itself, uncover its defect, and work on treatment and repair.

There are immediate clinical applications of this new marker for the HD gene. In families in which the marker is definitely linked to the gene, G8 can be used to detect the HD gene presymptomatically and prenatally, with 95 percent certainty. It is possible, however, that there is genetic heterogeneity in this illness as in most other hereditary diseases, and that some families may have their mutant gene on another chromosome. HD families from widely varying racial and ethnic backgrounds are currently being tested to determine if they, too, show linkage to G8. Different haplotypes of the marker are linked to the gene in the families studied, indicating that the marker is still some distance from the gene.

Once the question of genetic heterogeneity is resolved, the marker linkage test can be used clinically in appropriate families. It would be unethical to use it until heterogeneity information is collected. Presymptomatic and prenatal testing is an extraordinary boon for many HD families, but it also opens a Pandora's box of psychological, ethical, legal, and social questions. As there is no treatment, the outlook for those discovered to have the HD gene is bleak. The insidiousness of the first symptoms can cause years of protracted anxiety and anguish, stemming from uncertainty over whether symptoms have begun. The "sword of Damocles" thought to hang over those at risk is closer and more certain over the heads of presymptomatic individuals. How does one maintain health, love, commitment, and activity, knowing that the lethal gene may already be working its slow damage?

Even for those found to be free of risk, the information creates a radical upheaval in their self-images and identities. The "secondary gains" of being at-risk are lost, and life must be confronted with all options open.

The hiatus between our capacity to diagnose an at-risk person and treat an HD patient—to "liberate" someone from ambiguity to terror or joy with no other solace than excellent psychotherapy and support—will be one of psychological turmoil that we are presently ill equipped to handle. But the fact that we are confronted with this challenge is the most optimistic event in the history of HD research. We are closer to extracting the gene and learning its error—the crucial first step in designing rational and effective treatment. And the successful discovery of a marker for the HD gene using recombinant DNA techniques (the first time such techniques have localized a gene when the chromosomal assignment was unknown) pioneers this strategy for other hereditary diseases as well. As increasing numbers of RFLPs are discovered and the human genome is mapped, it should become successively easier to find genes of interest for Mendelian and polygenic disorders. The strategy being developed to find and correct the HD gene can be applied generally. But while science is preceding at an astonishing pace, there are awkward, interim phases in which all the skill, knowledge, and empathy of the mental health professions are required to cushion those affected until the next major breakthrough.

CONCLUSIONS

Lack of a predictive test, insidious symptom onset, multiple losses of family members, shifts in role responsibilities, increased financial burdens, loss of motor and cognitive capabilities with maintained insight, a terminal course—all these factors and others can keep HD families in conditions of chronic and prolonged stress, needing therapeutic intervention.

Rutter and colleagues, studying children from London's inner city and on the Isle of Wight, found that stresses potentiated each other and that "the combination of chronic stresses provided (very much) more than a summation of the effects of the separate stresses considered singly" (Wexler 1984). At Rockefeller University, Weiss is investigating the stress syndromes produced when one rat is "yoked" to another and receives exactly as many shocks as the partner but is unable to control receiving them. The yoked rat had almost four times the number of gastric lesions as the rat with the ability to exert control. (At the end of the experiment, the yoked animals looked, as close as animals can, depressed, becoming lethargic, and terminating eating, sleeping, and grooming behavior.) Weiss describes the factors leading to maximal stress: unpredictability, lack of control, and prolonged confinement in the stressful condition with no means of escape (Weiss 1980). An HD family fits all these criteria.

In Venezuela, they speak of all relatives of an HD patient as having inherited the illness, with only certain ones becoming sick. This medical fallacy expresses a psychological reality of ambiguity and threat, separate from the abnormal gene and passed on independently. As clinicians, our task should be to walk the border of neurology and psychiatry. As scientists, the eventual but certain decoding of the HD genetic error—however minuscule it may be—should clarify our understanding of feeling, thought, and motion from a novel perspective.

References

American Psychiatric Association: Diagnostic and Statistical Manual of Mental Disorders, 3rd ed. Washington, DC, American Psychiatric Association, 1980

Boehnke M, Conneally PM, Lange K: Two models for a maternal factor in the inheritance of Huntington's disease. Am J Hum Genet 35:845–860, 1983

Conneally PM: Huntington's disease: genetics and epidemiology. Am J Hum Genet 1984 (in press).

Folstein SE, Folstein MF: Psychiatric features of Huntington's disease. Psychol Dev 2:193–206, 1983

Folstein SE, Abbott MH, Chase GA, et al: The association of affective disorder with Huntington's disease in a case series and in families. Psychol Med 13:537–542, 1983

Gusella JF, Wexler NS, Conneally PM, et al: A polymorphic DNA marker genetically linked to Huntington's disease. Nature 306:234–238, 1983

Huntington G: On chorea. Med Surg Rep 26:317–321, 1872

Kuhl DE, Phelps ME, Markham CH, et al: Cerebral metabolism and atrophy in Huntington's disease determined by 18FDG and computed tomographic scan. Ann Neurol 12:425–434, 1982

Kurtzke JF: Huntington's disease: mortality and morbidity data from outside the United States, in Advances in Neurology, Vol 23: Huntington's Disease. Edited by Chase TN, Wexler NS, Barbeau A. New York, Raven Press, 1979

Spokes EG: Neurochemical alterations in Huntington's chorea. Brain 1:179–210, 1980

Weiss JM: Coping behavior: explaining behavioral depression following uncontrollable stressful events. Behav Res Ther 18:485–504, 1980

Wexler NS: Perceptual-motor, cognitive, and emotional characteristics of persons at risk for Huntington's disease, in Advances in Neurology, Vol 23: Huntington's Disease. Edited by Chase TN, Wexler NS, Barbeau A. New York, Raven Press, 1979, pp 239–255

Wexler NS: Huntington's disease and other late onset disorders, in Psychological Aspects of Genetic Counseling. Edited by Emory AE. London, Academic Press, 1984

4

Spontaneous Dyskinesias

Daniel E. Casey, M.D.
Thomas E. Hansen, M.D.

4

Spontaneous Dyskinesias

These movements remind one of choreic movements and are quite independent of ideas and feelings. (Kraepelin 1907, p 229)

In my entire, intensive and extensive experience I have never seen "choreal" disturbances which belong to schizophrenia. (Bleuler 1950, p 447)

Our ability to describe involuntary movement disorders far exceeds our capacity to explain them. While the narrative descriptions of dyskinesias over the last centuries retain a current relevance, the various hypothetical causes are much less useful and may even seem odd or naive because they were formulated in the context of beliefs prevalent at a given time. The earliest explanations involved superstitions of demonic possession, divinely or devilishly contrived punishment, overwhelming toxic substances, or generations of cursed family associations with evil.

We thank Marian K. Karr for expertly preparing the manuscript. This research was supported in part by funds from the Veterans Administration Research Career Development Award and Merit Review Program and NIMH grant no. 36657 (Dr. Casey).

Since these yet-to-be recognized syndromes of postinfectious, metabolic, hereditary, neurodegenerative, and psychotic disorders were often accompanied by personality changes, motor and mental abnormalities were inevitably and inextricably linked.

As physicians honed their observations to concise clinical descriptions, recognizable syndromes such as Parkinson's and Huntington's diseases (HD) were winnowed from the nondescript hodgepodge of movement disorders. Correlations between clinical signs and anatomical macro- and microscopic cerebral pathology further advanced the characterization of specific disorders. Unfortunately, the absence of demonstrable "organic" lesions has too often been used to verify the "functional" etiology of symptoms. This mind-body dualism is unnecessarily rigid and limits the theoretical flexibility needed to account for multiple determinations of complex syndromes. History teaches the lesson that many "functional" disorders of movement are eventually explained by improved understanding of "organic" central nervous system (CNS) function. It is a lesson that will undoubtedly be repeated with specific movement disorders.

One of the present-day controversies revolves around the issue of abnormal involuntary movements in psychiatric patients. The central question is whether neuroleptic drug treatment for psychosis plays a determinant role in causing hyperkinetic dyskinesias. On the surface, this seems like a straightforward statistical question to be answered simply by comparing rates of abnormal movements in patients before and after the onset of modern neuroleptic treatment in the 1950s. However, the matter is far more complex. It involves difficult questions of how to attribute proper weight to complex variables such as patient demographics, natural course of primary disease and intercurrent CNS dysfunction, influence of treatment, and consistency of symptom definition and assessment techniques.

A recurring theme in this review will be to address how much of the signs and symptoms of hyperkinetic dyskinesias should be attributed to the following factors: (1) chronic psychosis, particularly schizophrenia, (2) age-related CNS changes, and (3) treatment effects.

HISTORICAL BACKGROUND

Disagreements about the cause of disorders of movement in psychosis are not new. The controversy existed when Kraepelin and Bleuler were pioneering their formulations of schizophrenia (dementia praecox). Kraepelin, in the 1907 edition of his book *Clinical Psychiatry*, described signs that might be interpreted as findings similar to current-day drug-induced tardive dyskinesia (TD):

> There is still another type of convulsive movement, involving the muscles of the eye and speech, which is both characteristic and of frequent occurrence in dementia praecox. Some of these movements correspond exactly to the movements of expression: wrinkling of the eyebrow, distortion of the mouth, rolling the eyes, and those other facial movements which are characterized as grimacing. These movements remind one of choreic movements, and are quite independent of ideas and feelings. There may be associated with them smacking of the lips, clucking the tongue, sudden grunting, sniffing, and coughing. Furthermore, in the lips we observe very rapid rhythmical movements. More often there exists a peculiar choreiform movement of the mouth which may be described as an athetoid ataxia. (Kraepelin 1907, p 229)

In other revisions of this book and in his text *Dementia Praecox and Paraphrenia* (1919), Kraepelin variably decribed these signs as "spasmodic phenomena" that may be associated with "nystagmus" or "sudden laughing" and that "in no way bear the stamp of voluntary movements" (p 83).

Bleuler had a different view. In his discourse on mannerisms as accessory symptoms of psychosis, he stated:

> The expressive gestures are also modified. Every conceivable stilted gesture occurs. . . . Grimaces of all kinds, peculiar ways of shrugging the shoulder, extraordinary movements of tongue and lips, finger play, sudden involuntary gestures—all these peculiarities are the reason why some authors have spoken of choreic or tetanic movements in catatonia, quite mistakenly, though. (Bleuler 1950, p 191)

In the section of this text describing his theories of the motor symptoms of schizophrenia, Bleuler wrote:

> Choreal, athetotic, and tetanic phenomena are entirely different from the motor symptoms which accompany schizophrenia. (Bleuler 1950, p 445)

> In my entire, intensive and extensive experience I have never seen "choreal" disturbances which belong to schizophrenia. The reason why Wernicke's school assumes the presence of such disturbances, can only be that their concept of choreal movements extends far beyond anything which is actually seen in the various forms of chorea. The confinement of the movements to specific groups of muscles can be much better explained on a psychic than on an anatomic basis, aside from the fact that in some cases the psychic origin of the symptoms can be demonstrated. (Bleuler 1950, p 447)

How can we resolve these seemingly disparate points? Were Kraepelin and Bleuler seeing the same signs and symptoms, or were they recording fundamentally different observations about disorders of movement in schizophrenic patients? This question has no absolute answer. However, the most parsimonious explanation for the conflicting conclusions reached by these two astute observers centers around issues of definition of terms and theoretical framework. Both clinicians were probably describing similar phenomena but did not agree on terminology and etiology.

It is possible to argue that Kraepelin may have overinclusively tied together within a biological framework diverse and unrelated signs, whereas Bleuler may have too strictly conceptualized a psychological explanation for many abnormal movements. When evaluating "facial movements" and "grimacing," Kraepelin saw "chorea" and Bleuler saw "stereotypies and mannerisms." Such differences of diagnostic opinion continue as a present-day challenge.

The question is not whether these types of abnormal movements occurred prior to the drug treatment era. They surely did. Rather, it is a question of how much of what is now called "neuroleptic-induced TD" should actually be attributed to the natural history of psychosis, aging, or other nondrug causes.

EPIDEMIOLOGY

General Concerns

There are a number of shortcomings in the literature on spontaneous dyskinesias (SD). Useful information about such factors as age distribution, gender, psychiatric diagnosis, presence and type of organic mental syndrome, general state of health, and use of nonneuroleptic medication is frequently not reported. In comparisons of SD and drug-induced TD, chronically institution-alized, often elderly patients, with a variety of substantial disabil-ities, frequently are the only groups evaluated. Recently a few studies have addressed the issue of SD in noninstitutionalized patients, but the general lack of good studies is a cause for concern.

Since no single comprehensive nosology has been applied by investigators, the disorders studied were undoubtedly heteroge-neous. Whereas choreiform movements would be excluded in one study, tremor, stereotypies, and akathisia might be included as movement disorders in another. For instance, one report that specifically excluded stereotypy defined it in a manner that might include cases of typical orofacial dyskinesia:

> The most commonly observed stereotypies were rocking (18 patients), hand movements (19 patients), and oral movements (19 patients), the latter being lip smacking and munching, movements which were in themselves normal in appearance, but whose repetition constituted the abnormality. (Jones and Hunter 1969, p 54)

Just as the disorders studied were diverse, so too were the populations, which included patients of different ages with vary-ing degrees of organic mental disorders. Furthermore, well-recog-nized rating scales with defined criteria for symptom severity have been only occasionally used. Inclusion of all doubtful cases or only severe symptoms may have artifactually influenced rates of prevalence.

Prevalence

The prevalence rates of SD vary widely from 0 to 53.2 percent, with a weighted mean of 4.2 percent (Table 1). This value is consistent with those of other recent reviews that found mean prevalence rates of 5–7 percent (Smith and Baldessarini 1980; Jeste and Wyatt 1982; Kane and Smith 1982). These similarities assuredly reflect the substantial overlap of studies in each review.

Recognizing that substantial limitations in the data exist, we have summarized in Table 1 information from 24 reports of 29 samples involving 13,575 patients from divergent settings. To be included, reports only had to state how many patients not treated with neuroleptic medication had abnormal movements. Data from related studies by the same investigators evaluating dyskinesia rates in neuroleptic-treated patients are also included. Four reports (Degkwitz et al. 1967; Eckmann 1968; Heinrich et al. 1968; Hippius and Lange 1979) are cited secondarily from another paper (Kane and Smith 1982), as the original German articles were not reviewed.

One study conducted at a large state psychiatric institution prior to the first English language reports of TD and before neuroleptics were in general use found chorea and athetosis at the low prevalence rate of 0.6 percent in 5,704 patients (Mettler and Crandell 1959). Such a low rate is striking, as the authors expected a large number of neurological cases, and included 8 patients with HD (of the 35 with dyskinesia). One might speculate that only patients with severe disorders were counted as cases. On the other hand, the seemingly low prevalence may appear so only in the context of a trend where rates are higher in more recent reports on dyskinesias. Including this report with the other studies in Table 1 may bias the data, because the number of patients (5,704) examined was so large (43 percent of all patients reported). Excluding this study from the weighted mean changes the prevalence from 4.2 to 6.8 percent.

Prevalence rates for both SD and TD increase over time when data from studies that compare drugfree and drug-treated institutionalized patients are plotted (Figure 1). Previous authors con-

Table 1 Spontaneous and Tardive Dyskinesia Prevalence, 1959–1984

Study	Year	Spontaneous Dyskinesia		INST	Tardive Dyskinesia	
		Rate (%)	N		Rate (%)	N
Mettler and Crandell	1959	0.6	5,704	Yes	—	—
Demars	1966	6.8*	117	Yes	7.0	371
Siede and Müller	1967	1.2*	160	Yes	7.5	706
Degkwitz et al.	1967	1.4*	500	Yes	17.0	766
Degkwitz et al.	1967	0.9*	1,500	Yes	25.3	443
Degkwitz el al.	1967	1.5	912	Yes	—	—
Crane	1968	0	97	Yes	13.8	138
Heinrich et al.	1968	2.0	100	Yes	17.0	554
Heinrich et al.	1968	3.0	201	Yes	—	—
Eckmann	1968	4.1	613	Yes	2.9	828
Greenblatt et al.	1968	2.0*	101	Yes	38.4	52
Jones and Hunter	1969	2.2	45	Yes	20.7	82
Hippius and Lange	1970	13.9	137	Yes	34.3	531
Brandon et al.	1971	19.3	285	Yes	25.1	625
Crane	1973	2.0	46	Yes	15.7	1,324
Crane	1973	0*	28	Yes	17.9	56
Crane and Smeets	1974	25.0*	8	Yes	51.6	31
Delwaide and Desseilles	1977	36.7*	240	Yes	—	—
Bourgeois et al.	1980	18.0*	211	Yes	42.3	59
Kane et al.	1980	3.0	32	No	4.6	239
Blowers et al.	1981	31.7*	378	Yes	48.4	122
Owens et al.	1982	53.2	47	Yes	67.0	364
Kane et al.	1982	3.9*	127	No	—	—
Klawans and Barr	1982	5.0*	661	No	—	—
Jeste and Wyatt	1982	4.5	198	Yes	23.9	88
Varga et al.	1982	10.3*	340	Mixed	—	—
Barnes et al.	1983	11.8*	85	No	53.0	182
Lieberman et al.	1984	1.2*	400	No	—	—
Lieberman et al.	1984	4.8*	291	Yes	16.5	79

NOTE. N = number in overall population screened; INST = institutionalized patients.
* Elderly sample (aged >60 years or identifiable subpopulation over 60 years old).

cluded that the rise in TD did not primarily reflect increased interest or more sensitive examination methods (Jeste and Wyatt 1982; Kane and Smith 1982). However, these reports did not compare changes in prevalence rates of SD. Although such analyses must be done cautiously to avoid comparing highly dissimilar groups, this risk is moderated in the 19 studies (1966–1984) in Figure 1 because only reports of untreated and drug-treated patients who were evaluated by the same investigators are

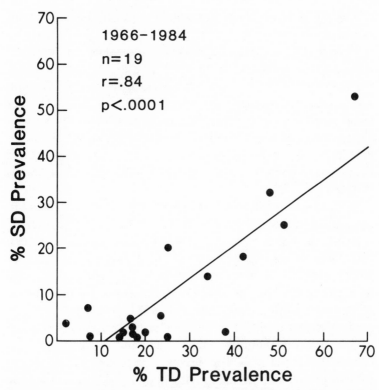

Figure 1 Prevalence of spontaneous dyskinesia (SD) and tardive dyskinesia (TD) in reports in which comparative populations were studied by the same investigators.

cited. The high correlation ($r = .84$, $p < .0001$) between the reported rates of SD and TD indicates that the prevalence rates of these disorders have increased proportionately over this period. This suggests that increased vigilance may have had a generalized effect on the reported rates of many types of dyskinesias. Whether "true" prevalence rates, estimated by Kane and Smith (1982) to be 5 percent for SD and 20 percent for TD, are actually changing remains an open question that must be addressed within the context of increasing awareness of movement disorders. However, the high correlation between the reported rates of these dyskinesias supports the argument that the relative prevalence of neuroleptic-induced TD is approximately 15 percent higher than that of SD.

Though the majority of reports demonstrate an increased prevalence of dyskinesia in drug-treated patients, a few do not (Table 1). One of these studies was not age-matched; the TD group was 10 years younger than the SD group (Demars 1966). Another report finding no drug effect did show a trend toward increased TD that was just below standard statistical significance ($p < .055$; Brandon et al. 1971). Reexamination of their data does show a significant drug effect in patients older than 50 ($\chi^2 = 13.44$, $df = 1$, $p < .011$).

A third study claiming no significant differences between prevalence rates of SD (53.2 percent) and TD (approximately 67 percent) also was not age matched but deserves special consideration because reliable rating scales with defined standards for severity were used (Owens et al. 1982). When these patients were matched for age, the prevalence of dyskinesia in the drug-treated group was significantly higher ($p < .05$) than in the untreated group (Crow et al. 1982). Medication status must also be considered before concluding that treated and untreated groups have similar dyskinesia rates. For instance, 79 percent of the treated patients in this study were receiving neuroleptic drugs at the time of evaluation (Owens et al. 1982), quite possibly masking some cases of TD. This discussion does not negate the finding of a high prevalence rate in untreated, debilitated, elderly, chronically institutionalized, schizophrenic patients. Rather, it underscores the importance of knowing what group of patients is studied under specified conditions.

Risk Factors

Age. SD rates increase with age. The few studies addressing this question across a broad age range found a positive correlation (Brandon et al. 1971; Klawans and Barr 1982; Barnes et al. 1983), as has also been shown with TD (Smith and Baldessarini 1980; Jeste and Wyatt 1982; Kane and Smith 1982). A fourth report did not find an age effect, but failed to include any patients younger than

60 years (Delwaide and Desseilles 1977).

A separate and less specific approach is to compare prevalence rates from studies involving patients whose mean age was greater than 60 years with the rates from the remaining studies in Table 1. Since many reports do not specify the ages of their population or identify the elderly patients, the nongeriatric group undoubtedly includes some patients over 60 years old. However, this will conservatively bias the data to increase the nongeriatric age and diminish differences between the groups. The geriatric prevalence rate is 7.7 percent, compared with 5.6 percent in the nongeriatric group, after excluding the sample of 5,704 patients noted previously ($\chi^2 = 12.08$, $df = 1$, $p = 5.1 \times 10^{-4}$; Mettler and Crandel 1959). This result is even more striking if the nongeriatric data of Mettler and Crandell are included for an SD prevalence of 2.3 percent ($\chi^2 = 223.55$, $df = 1$, $p = 1.5 \times 10^{-50}$).

Gender. Females are more often affected by SD than are males—a finding also reported with TD (1.68:1 ratio; Kane and smith 1982). Studies that divide prevalence rate data by sex present ratios of 1:1 (Degkwitz et al. 1967), 2.4:1 (Brandon et al. 1971), 2.9:1 (Delwaide and Desseilles 1977), and 1.8:1 (Klawans and Barr 1982). An additional study found only women affected (Demars 1966).

Institutionalization. Institutionalized patients (Table 1) have significantly higher SD prevalence rates (7.5 vs. 4.4 percent) than noninstitutionalized patients ($\chi^2 = 16.48$, $df = 1$, $p = 4.9 \times 10^{-5}$). The data from Mettler and Crandell (1959) are excluded because they constituted 74 percent of the institutionalized patients. If this study is included, there is no significant effect of institutionalization ($\chi^2 = .09$, $df = 1$, $p = 0.76$). When only geriatric population studies are examined, the differences in SD prevalence rates between institutionalized (8.5 percent) and noninstitutionalized (5.0 percent) are also significant ($\chi^2 = 14.10$, $df = 1$, $p = 1.7 \times 10^{-4}$). For the nongeriatric group, the effect of institutionalization (6.0 vs. 2.6 percent) is less obvious, though still statistically significant ($\chi^2 = 5.68$, $df = 1$, $p = 0.017$). If the data of Mettler and Crandell are included with the institutionalized nongeriatric data, no significant differences exist (2.2 vs. 2.6 percent).

Recent studies in which the reference population was not psychiatrically ill or institutionalized report much lower SD rates, ranging from 1 to 12 percent (Kane et al. 1982; Klawans and Barr 1982; Barnes et al. 1983; Lieberman et al. 1984).

Organic Mental Syndromes. The relationship between organic mental disorders and SD is difficult to evaluate. Some studies reported (Table 1) described reference populations with an increased likelihood of CNS disorders (patients from "senile wards" or "psychogeriatric units" or with specified prevalence rates for organic disorders). Recognizing that such a general categorization has substantial limitations, the dyskinesia prevalence rate for patients with and without organic mental disorders is 12.5 and 5.6 percent, respectively [$x^2 = 60.17$, $df = 1$, $p = 8.7 \times 10^{-15}$; Mettler and Crandell data (1959) excluded]. If organic mental disorders are borne out by more rigorous studies to be risk factors for SD, the same may eventually be confirmed for TD and influence the decision to prescribe neuroleptics to those at risk.

Medical Disorders. Medical disorders have received little attention as indicators for increased risk of SD. One recent study demonstrates a fourfold increase in prevalence for a medically ill and institutionalized elderly population (4.8 percent) compared with healthy elderly people (1.2 percent; Lieberman et al. 1984). Another study of noninstitutionalized patients with various medical problems found a prevalence (5 percent) similar to that for the above "medical" group (Klawans and Barr 1982). These findings again emphasize the need to define what population is studied when determining dyskinesia prevalence rates.

Meige's Syndrome

Meige's syndrome, originally described as "median facial spasm," consists of blepharospasm and oromandibular dystonia (Meige 1910). Though it is thought to be uncommon and not specifically associated with psychiatric illnesses, many cases re-

ported as spontaneous orofacial dyskinesias may have been examples of this syndrome (Appenzeller and Biehl 1968; Altrocchi
1972; Pakkenberg and Fog 1974). A recent report covering 100
patients also summarized 94 cases previously reported by others
(Jankovic and Ford 1983). Females constituted 62 percent of the
patients, similar to the ratio of females to males for SD noted above
(1.6:1). The mean age was 52 years (range 16–75 years), with the
number of afflicted patients increasing up to the seventh decade of
life. These results closely parallel findings in an early report of 135
patients with essential blepharospasm (Henderson 1956).

Conclusions

Methodologic problems in reports about SD limit our ability to
draw firm conclusions about the epidemiology of these disorders.
One must consider what population is being studied, predisposing
risk factors, diagnosis, and the time frame of the study, since
reported prevalence rates have risen over the last 25 years. The
overall rate of 4.2 percent includes low frequencies in otherwise
healthy populations (1–5 percent) but increases, possibly up to 50
percent, with the complex interaction among the additional risk
factors of increasing age, institutionalization, and organic mental
disorders in chronically ill psychiatric patients.

CLINICAL FEATURES

Definition and Description

Spontaneous dyskinesias constitute a heterogeneous group of
broadly defined abnormal involuntary movements that occur
along the continuum from chorea to athetosis to dystonia. Reports
have included movements of the face, with increased blinking
rates, blepharospasm, tongue movements or protrusion, lateral or
vertical jaw movements, and/or chewing motions; the trunk; and
the extremities, with choreoathetotic jerky and/or writhing
movements. Though studies have tended to include diverse
symptoms, it is not clear if orofacial and extremity dyskinesias are

part of the same disease process. Tremors should not be included in this class of SD.

Symptoms of stereotypies and mannerisms, commonly seen in schizophrenia, catatonia, and other psychoses, challenge the development of a coherent description of SD. Stereotypies are repetitive, purposeless movements that are often more complex than dyskinesia, and mannerisms are atypical of bizarre ways of carrying out purposeful activities that might be normal in some contexts. They may appear to be under voluntary control. Though on paper stereotypies and mannerisms seem distinct from dyskinesias like chorea, in practice they can be difficult to distinguish from each other.

Use of a broad definition for choreoathetosis and the limitations inherent in attributing psychologic meanings to bizarre behavior contribute to these difficulties. Stereotypies and mannerisms may be particularly common in catatonia, as prevalence rates of 26 (Morrison 1973) and 71 (Abrams and Taylor 1976) percent have been reported.

Differential Diagnosis

The differential diagnosis of SD includes a broad spectrum of idiopathic, drug-induced, hereditary, and associated neuromedical conditions.

Idiopathic Dyskinesias. Differentiating stereotypic and manneristic behavior in patients with chronic psychosis is often difficult (see above). Meige's syndrome (blepharospasm and oromandibular dystonia) must be distinguished from other focal and segmental dystonias (Marsden 1976). Tourette's syndrome (TS) is a disorder of involuntary tics and vocalizations that starts in childhood and continues with a waxing and waning course through adult life (see Chapter 2). Simple persisting tics in an isolated muscle group must also be recognized. Dental problems with caries, gum disease, or poorly fitting dentures can cause orofacial movements, but are not associated with any extremity dyskinesias (Sutcher et al. 1971).

Drug-induced Dyskinesias. TD, which may appear identical to many signs of SD, should not be diagnosed, with rare exception, in patients who have had fewer than three months of neuroleptic treatment (see Chapter 5). Though the term "TD" is often loosely applied to many descriptions, it should be restricted to the specific identification of neuroleptic-induced dyskinesias. Anticholinergic agents have occasionally produced orofacial and limb dyskinesias after prolonged use, and chronic antihistamine use has rarely been associated with such symptoms. Amphetamines can produce dyskinesias as well as stereotyped behavior. Phenytoin and other anticonvulsants can produce reversible orofacial dyskinesias, as can oral contraceptives. Levodopa produces dyskinesias similar to TD and SD, but this drug is used primarily in Parkinson's disease. Chloroquine and other antimalarial drugs can also produce pronounced facial dyskinesias (Casey 1981).

Hereditary Neurodegenerative and Systemic Illnesses. The hereditary neurodegenerative diseases such as HD (see Chapter 3), Wilson's disease (hepatolenticular degeneration associated with metabolic disorders of copper metabolism), and Hallervorden-Spatz syndrome (disorder of iron metabolism) may initially present with signs that resemble SD. These syndromes are usually distinguishable by clinical signs, laboratory tests, family history, and the course of the illness. Endocrinopathies such as hyperthyroidism or hypoparathyroidism, systemic lupus erythematosus, chorea in pregnancy (chorea gravidarum), and postinfectious CNS syndromes can all be associated with involuntary movements.

Course and Prognosis

Only rudimentary knowledge about the course and prognosis of SD exists. Though many patients have only mild symptoms with little or no disability, it has been suggested that orofacial dyskinesia can be an early manifestation of generalized "senile" chorea (Weiner and Klawans 1973). Meige's syndrome usually has a gradual onset and stabilizes after several years with impairment ranging from mild to severe (Jankovic and Ford 1983). The presence of dyskinesias in schizophrenia may be correlated with poor prognosis (Kraepelin 1970; Yarden and Discipio 1971).

Rating Scales

A variety of rating scales have been developed for abnormal involuntary movements. Although any of these can be used for SD, the Abnormal Involuntary Movement Scale is well suited owing to its simple design that rates movements by body part and for overall severity (Guy 1976).

The literature on SD would become more easily interpreted if investigators applied the same criteria. Utilizing the research diagnostic criteria proposed for TD would greatly improve our ability to compare dyskinetic disorders (Schooler and Kane 1982). These criteria require at least moderate involvement of one body area or mild symptoms in two or more areas, and assess the temporal stability of the movements (transient versus probable or persistent dyskinesia).

ETIOLOGY AND NEUROPATHOLOGY

The causes of SD are unknown. Recent research has focused on identifying age-related CNS changes, particularly in the basal ganglia and in the neurotransmitters dopamine (DA) and acetylcholine. This interest has been stimulated by advancements in our understanding of Parkinson's disease, another age-related movement disorder (see Chapter 1). Though Parkinson's disease is characterized by an absolute decrease of DA, leading to a relative overfunction of acetylcholine, the pathophysiology of SD is unclear. Treatment approaches to SD have centered on a purported overfunction of DA and acetylcholine, although a deficit of the latter has also been posited.

Alterations in DA function have been the ones most studied. Brain DA levels decrease with increasing age (Carlsson 1976), and enzymes that deactivate DA, such as monoamine oxidase and catechol-O-methyltransferase, increase with age (Robinson et al. 1971; Smith and Leelavathi 1980). Decreased DA levels might lead to biochemical "denervation supersensitivity," as has been proposed as a pathophysiological mechanism underlying TD. This should lead to a compensatory increase in DA receptor function. However, the data do not support this line of reasoning to explain SD. DA-stimulated adenylcyclase and receptor binding to DA antagonists show a decrease in receptor numbers with increasing age (Makman et al. 1979; Pradhan 1980), but receptor binding to DA agonists shows little change (DiBlasi et al. 1982). Behavioral studies show an increased response to both DA agonists, as measured by stereotypic behavior, and DA antagonists, as measured by catalepsy (Smith et al. 1978; Campbell et al. 1984). These increased responses may be due to an actual increase in the sensitivity of the CNS or to some other age-related changes such as reduced drug metabolism (Campbell et al. 1984). In another study with rats, no differences in receptor numbers were found that could explain the different rates of perioral movements in drug-treated and control animals (Crow et al. 1982).

Neuropathological data are sparse. One evaluation in a small number of patients reported striatal cell loss in "senile" chorea (Alcock 1936). Another study comparing the postmortem findings between patients with SD and those with TD found substantial cell loss and gliosis in both groups, though the findings were more prevalent in the TD group (Christensen et al. 1970). The study reporting similar rates of SD and TD in chronic schizophrenic patients (Owens et al. 1982) found no differences in the postmortem evaluation of DA receptors that correlated with the presence or absence of abnormal movements (Crow et al. 1982).

ANIMAL MODELS

The absence of an animal model limits potential research in SD. One novel approach has been to apply to nonhuman primates the cross-sectional epidemiologic model of investigation most commonly used in the studies of the prevalence of SD and drug-induced TD.

In a study with 227 rhesus monkeys (aged 1–28 years), spontaneously occurring orofacial dyskinesias were assessed (Casey 1982).

Two different levels of symptom frequency were established to define a case of SD: symptoms were present occasionally (10 percent—mild) or continuously (100 percent—severe).

Spontaneous dyskinesias occurred at low prevalence levels for the first 15 years of life, but then increased in those over 16 years old. Prevalence rates varied widely, depending on two factors: the criteria set to define a case, and the size of the base population used as a denominator for subjects at risk. If the highest criterion (100 percent) was used, only 1 of 227 monkeys (prevalence 0.4 percent) had SD. The other extreme was to evaluate the lowest criterion (10 percent) of symptoms in the monkeys most at risk (>20 years old). In this latter case, 10 of 41 monkeys (prevalence 24.4 percent) qualified for a diagnosis of SD. Intermediate prevalence rates occurred between these points, depending on symptom frequency and population at risk.

Spontaneous dyskinesias, such as tongue protrusion and chewing symptoms that are identical to those in humans, occur in nonhuman primates. The prevalence is relatively low in younger and midadult life, and then increases when monkeys are older than 16 years. Converting rhesus monkey age to human age (approximately 1:3.5 years), the primary increase in SD occurs when monkeys are at the equivalent age of 55 human years. These findings are consistent with the observations that both SD and TD occur more commonly with advancing age.

The prevalence rate of SD is strikingly dependent upon the criteria used for defining a case. The strictest criteria have the lowest prevalence rate of 0.4 percent, whereas the least stringent criteria have prevalence rates of 24.4 percent. This range, which approximates the findings in the human studies cited above, emphasizes the point that the existing reports were strongly influenced by experimental design issues related to symptom severity, types and number of patients studied, and age ranges.

Spontaneous dyskinesias in monkeys, and possibly in aged rodents, suggest that there is a naturally occurring low base rate of these symptoms. With advancing age there may also be an increasing vulnerability within the individual to develop SD. Exposure to elements that increase the likelihood of converting a covert predisposition to overt symptoms will depend on multiple factors; extended neuroleptic treatment may be just one of these. This view is consistent with the findings cited above that note an approximate 4–5 percent rate of SD and a 20 percent rate of drug-induced TD. Whereas the absolute values of and differences between SD and TD prevalence rates are arguable, the pattern of relative difference remains.

MANAGEMENT AND TREATMENT

Systematic studies of the management and treatment of SD are noticeably lacking. Most reports involve only small numbers of patients with Meige's syndrome or other focal dystonias treated during open therapeutic trials. Therefore, these sketchy treatment results should not necessarily be generalized to patients with long-term psychiatric or neurological illnesses. If psychosis is present, evaluating and treating this condition should take priority.

The treatment strategy should be formulated within the context of symptom evolution and severity. Most cases of SD develop slowly over many months to years. Some patients are minimally aware of their symptoms, but others are greatly troubled by social embarrassment and/or physical discomfort if painful muscle spasms are present. A differential diagnosis and evaluation of potentially treatable causes of dyskinesias should be followed by a series of pharmacological trials, if symptoms are severe enough to warrant treatment. Surgical interventions should be reserved for severe and incapacitating symptoms. Psychological and behavioral therapies may be useful adjuncts, but there is little support for these approaches as the primary or sole form of treatment.

Many different pharmacological approaches have been tried in an attempt to control SD, but no one medication has been uniformly effective. Drugs that benefit one patient may have no effect on or may aggravate symptoms in another. Antagonists and agonists of DA and acetylcholine, the principal pharmacologic approaches to other movement disorders, have been most commonly used, though drugs influencing other monoamines (e.g., norepinephrine) and γ-aminobutyric acid (GABA) have also been tried (Marsden 1976; Delwaide and Desseilles 1977; Tolosa and Lai 1979; Casey 1980; Jankovic and Ford 1983; Casey 1984). The absence of a predictable and uniform treatment outcome further emphasizes the probable heterogeneity of the pathophysiological mechanisms underlying clinically similar disorders.

Dopaminergic predominance in the basal ganglia is a purported pathophysiological mechanism underlying SD, particularly in Meige's syndrome (Tolosa and Lai 1979). Neuroleptic drugs may partially decrease symptoms, but often at the expense of developing unacceptable drug-induced parkinsonism. A strategy to decrease DA function akin to neuroleptic-induced receptor blockade can be achieved by depleting presynaptic DA with reserpine (Jankovic and Ford 1983). However, a major caution must be raised. It is possible that suppressing symptoms with prolonged drug treatment that inhibits DA function will eventually aggravate or cause TD, though there are no firm data to substantiate this concern. If neuroleptic drugs are required for severe symptoms, they may be effective at relatively low doses, such as chlorpromazine (Thorazine) 50–400 mg/day or haloperidol (Haldol) 1–8 mg/day. Reserpine must be started at low doses and slowly built up to 0.5–2.0 mg/day. Potential problems of hypotension, nasal stuffiness, and depression are important concerns.

Conversely, DA agonists such as carbidopa/levodopa (Sinemet), amantadine (Symmetrel), and bromocriptine (Parlodel) have been used. Again, no outcome is predictable, though many patients will have their symptoms increase with these compounds.

Trials with anticholinergic compounds have also produced conflicting results. Trihexyphenidyl (Artane), benztropine (Cogentin), and other anticholinergics and antihistaminic drugs such as orphenadrine (Norflex) and diphenhydramine (Benadryl) have provided symptomatic improvement for some patients and no benefit or worsening in others. Recently recommended high-dose anticholinergic drugs, particularly for Meige's syndrome or some related dyskinetic/dystonic disorders (Fahn 1983), should be used cautiously because of anticholinergic toxicity.

Cholinergic agonists have also been evaluated. Physostigmine often aggravates symptoms, suggesting possible overfunction of cholinergic mechanisms, which is consistent with the beneficial findings of anticholinergic agents. Physostigmine, however, is not for routine use or evaluation, and should be reserved for experimental trials because of its potent effects. Cholinergic precursors such as choline and lecithin are of theoretical interest, but there are insufficient data to support a recommendation for this treatment approach.

A wide selection of other pharmacological approaches has been tried with variable results. These include antidepressants, such as amitriptyline (Elavil) and imipramine (Tofranil), the serotonergic benzodiazepine anticonvulsant clonazepam (Clonapin) and the antispastic GABA analog baclofen (Lioresal), and the antianxiety agents diazepam (Valium) and chlordiazepoxide (Librium). In all cases, these and other drug treatments are considered palliative and aimed at symptomatic control. No medications have been curative and none is specifically indicated for the treatment of SD.

Taking a pharmacologic approach to these symptoms is time consuming and potentially fraught with frustration. Indeed, after many months of drug trials, no medication may turn out to be effective. This approach requires patience on behalf of both the patient and the physician, because of disappointments and intolerance to drug side effects.

Psychotherapeutically supportive treatments may be useful for patients who are understandably frustrated and have difficulty making adjustments in their life-style. Many patients become depressed at some time during attempts to deal with their symptoms. If depression is serious, antidepressant medication and/or psychotherapy is indicated. If the patient is psychotic, appropriate drug therapy should be used.

A psychological etiology of SD has been hypothesized for decades, but there is no convincing evidence to support this proposal or to document the therapeutic value of insight-oriented psychotherapy. If psychotherapy is indicated, the focus should be on helping patients adapt to the limitations imposed by their symptoms. Behavior therapy and biofeedback may also be beneficial in selected cases, though the long-term outcome of this treatment approach is unknown. These psychotherapeutic approaches are aimed at providing patients with some control over their symptoms and should not imply a psychologic origin of the disorder.

Surgery for SD should be considered as an option only for the most severe symptoms in well-selected cases. Surgical techniques aimed at severe blepharospasm or intolerable symptoms of oromandibular dystonia have focused on peripheral intervention of the facial nerve. Because there is variable and collateral innervation of the affected muscles, the outcome is unpredictable and there is the possibility of reinnervation with a high rate of symptom recurrence. Surgical lesioning of the CNS, such as thalamotomy, is not recommended, and should be reserved for only the most severe crippling dyskinesias.

SUMMARY

One of the current controversies in psychiatry centers around the issue of involuntary movement disorders. It is not a question of whether all dyskinesias are drug related. Surely they are not, since these types of disorders were well described prior to the modern era of neuroleptic treatment. Debate about the causes of these disorders also is not new. Kraepelin and Bleuler described similar SD phenomena but disagreed on terminology and hypothesized conflicting explanations. The question to answer is: How much of what is now called "neuroleptic-induced TD" is actually SD and should be more properly attributed to the natural history of psychosis, aging, or other nondrug causes?

Though substantial methodological differences exist among the reports about the epidemiology of SD, some general patterns emerge. The overall prevalence rate is 4.2 percent, but includes low frequencies in otherwise healthy populations (1–5 percent) and high rates, possibly up to 50 percent, in more vulnerable groups. Risk factors for SD include increasing age, institutionalization, and underlying CNS dysfunction.

Reported prevalence rates for both SD and TD have increased over the last 20 years in studies of institutionalized patients. However, these increases have been approximately proportional and continue to show that the prevalence of TD is about 15 percent higher than that of SD. Perhaps with advancing age there is an increasing vulnerability to develop naturally occurring SD. Exposure to extended neuroleptic treatment is one of the factors that enhance the likelihood of converting a covert predisposition to overt symptoms.

In a study evaluating the rates of SD across a wide range of ages in rhesus monkeys, the prevalence rate increased with age. However, the absolute value for the rate varied widely, depending on two factors: the criteria set to define a case and the size of the base population used as a denominator for subjects at risk. With the strictest criterion, the prevalence rate was only 0.4 percent, but with the most relaxed criterion, the prevalence was 24.4 percent. These findings clearly demonstrate that prevalence rates in clinical populations must be interpreted within the context of criteria for defining a case, the age and size of the population at risk, instruments used for assessment, and which patients are being studied (e.g., healthy versus aged institutionalized patients).

Spontaneous dyskinesias, which closely resemble the signs and symptoms of TD, encompass a broad differential diagnosis. This includes the idiopathic hyperkinetic dyskinesias of stereotypic and manneristic behavior of psychosis, Meige's syndrome, other focal or segmental dystonias, TS, simple tics, and dental problems. Additional distinctions must be made among drug-induced dyskinesias, hereditary neurodegenerative disorders, and dyskinesias associated with systemic neuromedical illnesses. The causes of SD are unknown, and there are no confirmed neuropathological findings in this disorder.

Treatment of SD has been insufficiently studied. Most of the reports involved small numbers of patients who did not have long-term psychiatric illnesses, but who suffered from such idiopathic disorders as Meige's syndrome. Dopaminergic antagonists are the most effective drugs for suppressing SD, but trials with cholinergic, GABAergic, noradrenergic blocking, serotonergic, and other compounds have been variably effective. However, there is the continuing concern that suppressing SD with pharmacotherapy may eventually lead to its aggravation or to the development of

TD. No data exist to support the rationale of treating SD solely with psychotherapeutic approaches, though these techniques may be useful adjuncts for assisting patients to adapt to their symptoms. Surgical approaches to SD should be reserved for only the severest symptoms in carefully selected patients after other treatment approaches have failed.

Future directions for research should focus on the epidemiology, etiology, and treatment of SD. Methodological improvements with increasing control of relevant variables will greatly assist our study of these disorders. Ideally, prospective studies should be done to clarify important differences between SD and TD.

References

Abrams R, Taylor MA: Catatonia, a prospective clinical study. Arch Gen Psychiatry 33:579–581, 1976

Alcock NS: A note on the pathology of senile chorea (non-hereditary). Brain 59:376–387, 1936

Altrocchi PH: Spontaneous oral-facial dyskinesia. Arch Neurol 26:506–512, 1972

Appenzeller O, Biehl JP: Mouthing in the elderly: a cerebellar sign. J Neurol Sci 6:249–260, 1968

Barnes TRE, Rosser M, Trauer T: A comparison of purposeless movements in psychiatric patients treated with antipsychotic drugs and normal individuals. J Neurol Neurosurg Psychiatry 46:540–546, 1983

Bleuler E: Dementia Praecox or the Group of Schizophrenias. 1911 ed. Translated by Zinkin J. New York, International Universities Press, 1950

Blowers AJ, Borison RL, Blowers CM, et al: Abnormal involuntary movements in the elderly. Br J Psychiatry 139:363–364, 1981

Bourgeois M, Bouilh P, Tignol J, et al: Spontaneous dyskinesias versus neuroleptic-induced dyskinesias in 270 elderly subjects. J Nerv Ment Dis 168:177–178, 1980

Brandon S, McClelland HA, Protheroe C: A study of facial dyskinesia in a mental hospital population. Br J Psychiatry 118:171–184, 1971

Campbell A, Baldessarini RJ, Stoll A, et al: Effect of age on behavioral responses and tissue levels of apomorphine in the rat. Neuropharmacology 1984 (in press)

Carlsson A: Some aspects of dopamine in the basal ganglia, in The Basal Ganglia. Edited by Yahr MD. New York, Raven Press, 1976, pp 181–189

Casey DE: Pharmacology of blepharospasm-oromandibular dystonia syndrome. Neurology 30:690–695, 1980

Casey DE: The differential diagnosis of tardive dyskinesia. Acta Psychiatr Scand 63 (suppl 291):71–87, 1981

Casey DE: Spontaneous orofacial dyskinesias in rhesus monkeys: age-related prevalence rates. Proc Soc Biol Psychiatry 100:131, 1982

Casey DE: Essential blepharospasm, in Current Ocular Therapy. Philadelphia, WB Saunders, 1984 (in press)

Christensen E, Møller JE, Faurbye A: Neuropathological investigation of 28 brains from patients with dyskinesia. Acta Psychiatr Scand 46:14–23, 1970

Crane GE: Dyskinesia and neuroleptics. Arch Gen Psychiatry 19:700–703, 1968

Crane GE: Persistent dyskinesia. Br J Psychiatry 122:395–405, 1973

Crane GE, Smeets RA: Tardive dyskinesia and drug therapy in geriatric patients. Arch Gen Psychiatry 30:341–343, 1974

Crow TJ, Cross AJ, Johnstone EC, et al: Abnormal involuntary movements in schizophrenia: are they related to the disease process or to its treatment? Are they associated with changes in dopamine receptors? J Clin Psychopharmacol 2:336–340, 1982

Degkwitz R, Binsack KF, Herkert H, et al: Zum Problem der persistieren den extrapyramidalen Hyperkinesen nach langfristiger Anwendung von Neuroleptika. Nervenarzt 38:170–174, 1967

Delwaide PJ, Desseilles M: Spontaneous buccolingualfacial dyskinesia in the elderly. Acta Neurol Scand 56:256–262, 1977

Demars JCA: Neuromuscular effects of long-term phenothiazine medication, electroconvulsive therapy, and leucotomy. J Nerv Ment Dis 143:73–79, 1966

DiBlasi A, Cotecchia S, Mennini T: Selective changes of receptor binding in brain regions of aged rats. Life Sci 31:335–340, 1982

Eckmann F: Zur Problematik von Dauerschäden nach neuroleptischer Langzeitbehandlung. Ther Ggw 107:316–323, 1968

Fahn S: High dosage anticholinergic therapy in dystonia. Neurology 33:1255–1261, 1983

Greenblatt DL, Dominick JR, Stotsky BA, et al: Phenothiazine-induced dyskinesia in nursing home patients. J Am Geriatr Soc 16:27–34, 1968

Guy W: ECDEU Assessment Manual for Psychopharmacology. Washington, DC, DHEW, 1976, pp 534–537

Heinrich K, Wegener I, Bender HJ: Späte extrapyramidale Hyperkinesen bei neuroleptischer Langzeit-Therapie. Pharmakopsychiatr Neuropsychopharmakol 1:161–195, 1968

Henderson JW: Essential blepharospasm. Trans Am Ophthalmol Soc 54:453–520, 1956

Hippius H, Lange J: Zur Problematik der späten extrapyramidelen Hyperkinesen nach langfristiger neuroleptischer Therapie. Arzneim Forsch 20:88–890, 1970

Jankovic J, Ford J: Blepharospasm and orofacial-cervical dystonia: clinical and pharmacologic findings in 100 patients. Ann Neurol 13:402–411, 1983

Jeste DV, Wyatt RJ: Understanding and Treating Tardive Dyskinesia. New York, Guilford, 1982, pp 15–20, 33–34

Jones M, Hunter R: Abnormal movements in patients with chronic psychiatric illness, in Psychotropic Drugs and Dysfunctions of the Basal Ganglia. Edited by Crane GE, Gardner R. Washington, DC, Public Health Service publication no. 1938, 1969, pp 53–62

Kane JM, Smith JM: Tardive dyskinesia: prevalence and risk factors, 1959–1979. Arch Gen Psychiatry 39:473–481, 1982

Kane JM, Wegner J, Stenzler S, et al: The prevalence of presumed tardive dyskinesia in psychiatric inpatients and outpatients. Psychopharmacology 62:247–251, 1980

Kane JM, Weinhold P, Kinon B, et al: Prevalence of abnormal involuntary movements ("spontaneous dyskinesias") in the normal elderly. Psychopharmacology 77:105–108, 1982

Klawans HL, Barr A: Prevalance of spontaneous lingual-facial-buccal dyskinesias in the elderly. Neurology 32:558–559, 1982

Kraepelin E: Clinical Psychiatry. Adapted by Defendorf AR. New York, Macmillan, 1907

Kraepelin E: Dementia Praecox and Paraphrenia. 1919 ed. Translated by Barclay RM. Huntington, Krieger, 1971

Lieberman J, Kane J, Woerner M, et al: Prevalence of tardive dyskinesia in elderly samples. Psychopharmacol Bull 20:22–26, 1984

Makman MH, Ahn HS, Thal LM, et al: Aging and monoamine receptors in brain. Fed Proc 38:1922–1926, 1979

Marsden CD: Blepharospasm-oromandibular dystonia syndrome (Brueghel's syndrome). J Neurol Neurosurg Psychiatry 39:1204–1209, 1976

Meige H: Les convulsions de la face, une forme clinique de convulsion faciale, bilaterale et mediane. Rev Neurol (Paris) 2:437–443, 1910

Mettler FA, Crandell A: Neurologic disorders in psychiatric institutions. J Nerv Ment Dis 128:148–159, 1959

Morrison JR: Catatonia—retarded and excited types. Arch Gen Psychiatry 28:39–44, 1973

Owens DGC, Johnstone EC, Frith CD: Spontaneous involuntary disorders of movement. Arch Gen Psychiatry 39:452–461, 1982

Pakkenberg H, Fog R: Spontaneous oral dyskinesia. Arch Neurol 31:352–353, 1974

Pradhan SN: Central neurotransmitters and aging: mini-review. Life Sci 26:1643–1656, 1980

Robinson DS, Davis JM, Neese A, et al: Relations of sex and aging to monoamine oxidase activity of human brain, plasma and platelets. Arch Gen Psychiatry 24:536–639, 1971

Schooler N, Kane JM: Research diagnoses for tardive dyskinesia. Arch Gen Psychiatry 39:486–487, 1982

Seide H, Müller HF: Choreiform movements as side effects of phenothiazine medications in geriatric patients. J Am Geriatr Soc 15:517–522, 1967

Smith JM, Baldessarini RJ: Changes in prevalence, severity, and recovery in tardive dyskinesia with age. Arch Gen Psychiatry 37:1368–1373, 1980

Smith RC, Leelavathi DE: Behavioral and biochemical effects of chronic neuroleptic drugs: interaction with age, in Tardive Dyskinesia: Research and Treatment. Edited by Fann WE, Smith RC, Davis JM, et al. Jamaica, Spectrum, 1980, pp 65–88

Smith RC, Leelavathi DE, Lauritzen AM: Behavioral effects of dopamine agonists increase with age. Commun Psychopharmacol 2:39–43, 1978

Sutcher HD, Underwood RB, Beatty RA, et al: Orofacial dyskinesia, a dental dimension. JAMA 216:1459–1463, 1971

Tolosa ES, Lai CW: Meige disease: striatal dopaminergic preponderance. Neurology 29:1126–1130, 1979

Varga E, Sugerman AA, Varga V, et al: Prevalence of spontaneous oral dyskinesia in the elderly. Am J Psychiatry 139:329–331, 1982

Weiner WJ, Klawans HL: Lingual-facial-buccal movements in the elderly: II. Pathogenesis and relationship to senile chorea. J Am Geriatr Soc 21:318–320, 1973

Yarden PE, Discipio WJ: Abnormal movements and prognosis in schizophrenia. Am J Psychiatry 128:317–323, 1971

5

Tardive Dyskinesia

John M. Kane, M.D.
Margaret Woerner, Ph.D.
Jeffrey Lieberman, M.D.
Bruce Kinon, M.D.

5

Tardive Dyskinesia

Soon after the introduction of neuroleptics, it became apparent that these drugs were capable of producing a variety of extrapyramidal side effects, e.g., akinesia, rigidity, and acute dystonic reactions. These effects were observed to occur early in treatment, usually after days to weeks; to be transient, remitting spontaneously in some cases; generally to respond well to anticholinergic agents; and frequently but not always to disappear after neuroleptic dosage reduction or discontinuation.

Initial reports of tardive dyskinesia (TD) appeared in Europe in the late 1950s. Schonecker (1957) is generally credited with the first published description of TD in a paper entitled "A Peculiar Syndrome in Oral Region as a Result of the Administration of Megaphen." The three patients described with what may have been TD were elderly women, all of whom were said to have cerebral arteriosclerosis and who developed lip-smacking movements following a relatively brief exposure (2–8 weeks) to chlorpromazine. In two of the three, movements persisted for 4–11 weeks after discontinuation of chlorpromazine, and in the third, movements persisted for 12 weeks with continued chlorpromazine administration. Although these movements occurred earlier than what generally became associated with the concept of

Investigations described in this report were supported by NIMH grant MH 32369 and NIMH contract 278-82-0032.

"tardive" dyskinesia, the fact that they persisted following drug withdrawal suggested this was a different phenomenon from the previously recognized "parkinsonian" side effects.

Sigwald et al. (1959) provided the first detailed description of this condition and used the term "faciobuccolingual masticatory dyskinesia" to describe the movements observed in four elderly women who had been on neuroleptics for 3–18 months. The movements persisted for 6–27 months despite withdrawal of neuroleptics. In addition, these authors described three subtypes of neuroleptic-induced dyskinesias: acute, occurring early in treatment and remitting rapidly; subacute, occurring later in treatment and disappearing within 1–2 weeks of discontinuing the drug; and chronic, persisting long after the discontinuation of neuroleptics.

In 1960 Uhrbrand and Faurbye published the first report from an epidemiological perspective. They described 29 patients with buccolingual masticatory dyskinesia, including some patients who also had truncal and extremity involvement. Among 17 patients in whom the neuroleptic was discontinued, 11 had dyskinesia that persisted over a period ranging from 4 to 22 months. The authors also noted that some cases appeared for the first time or became worse upon neuroleptic withdrawal. They also suggested that elderly patients with "organic" brain disease were at particular risk for developing the condition for which they later (Faurbye et al. 1964) suggested the term "tardive dyskinesia."

Since these early reports, numerous epidemiologic studies have appeared, helping to put in better perspective the true scope and nature of the problem. In addition, several major books (Fann et al. 1980; Jeste and Wyatt 1982) and review articles (Jeste and Wyatt 1981; Kane and Smith 1982) as well as an American Psychiatric Association Task Force Report (Baldessarini et al. 1980) have helped to critique, integrate, and summarize existing knowledge as well as to point out unanswered questions and specific needs for future research.

CLINICAL FEATURES AND DIAGNOSIS

There are no pathognomonic signs or symptoms for the diagnosis of TD. It is not a diagnosis that can be made simply on the basis of a rating scale score or a physical examination. These procedures may indicate a high index of suspicion or a "presumptive" diagnosis, but additional steps are necessary to rule out other possible etiologies and to implicate, to the extent possible, neuroleptic drugs in the etiology. TD should be a diagnosis confined to a condition occurring in neuroleptic-treated patients, characterized by a variable mixture of orofacial dyskinesia, tics, facial grimacing, truncal or axial muscle involvement, chorea, athetosis, and dystonias. In addition, speech and respiration may also be affected.

The majority of surveys in the literature have suggested orofacial involvement to be by far the most frequent manifestation of TD. However, since this symptom pattern was originally considered the hallmark of TD, many cases without obvious orofacial movements may not have been included in some reports. It does appear, however, that among elderly individuals, the orofacial area is most frequently affected. This estimate may be inflated to some extent by the occurrence of "spontaneous" dyskinesias (SD; some of which might result from the edentulous state) occurring in non-neuroleptic-treated, elderly individuals.

It has been suggested that subsyndromes or subtypes of TD may be identified on the basis of bodily distribution, but further work is needed to validate this notion.

TD has been reported in children. Although the patterns of body distribution may vary, orofacial involvement is seen in some children, contrary to earlier notions (Gualtieri et al. 1982).

TD shares common features with some other movement disorders and choreoathetotic syndromes, in that movements may become worse with stress, diminish with sedation, and abate during sleep. This pattern is not consistent, however, and some individuals with TD may exhibit more movements during a relaxed state than during examination or close observation.

A diagnosis of TD should be entertained in any patient with abnormal involuntary movements, who has a history of taking neuroleptic medication for a period of at least 3 months. In many but not all cases, a drug dosage reduction or discontinuation may precede the onset of the movements. However, given the fact that neuroleptic drugs are capable of masking or suppressing some involuntary movement disorders besides TD, the emergence of movements under these circumstances should not preclude a careful differential diagnosis.

Table 1 lists differential diagnoses to be considered in evaluating a possible case of TD. The American Psychiatric Association Task Force Report (Baldessarini et al. 1980) suggested the following as a reasonable list of studies to be done in investigating a presumed case of TD: evaluation by a neurological consultant, chemistry profile, thyroid function studies, liver function tests, sedimentation rate, serum ceruloplasmin, urinary copper, electroencephalogram, and in selected cases a computed tomography scan. It has also been suggested that the diagnostic process in TD should involve a longitudinal perspective. Schooler and Kane (1982) have developed criteria for categorizing TD on the basis of serial

Table 1 Differential Diagnoses to Consider in Evaluating Tardive Dyskinesia

- Neuroleptic withdrawal-emergent dyskinesias or other transient acute dyskinesias associated with neuroleptics
- Late and persistent "classical" tardive dyskinesia itself*
- Stereotyped movements of schizophrenia*
- Spontaneous oral dyskinesias of advanced age or senility*
- Oral dyskinesias related to dental conditions or prostheses
- Idiopathic torsion dystonia
- Focal dystonias (oromandibular dystonia, blepharospasm, spasmodic torticollis) and "habit spasms" (tics)
- Huntington's disease*
- Gilles de la Tourette syndrome
- Wilson's disease (hepato-cerebral-lenticular degeneration owing to abnormal copper metabolism), manganism, and other heavy metal intoxications*
- Fahr's syndrome or other disorders with calcification of the basal ganglia
- Postanoxic, postencephalitic, encephalitic, or extrapyramidal syndromes*
- Rheumatic (Sydenham's) chorea ("St. Vitus' Dance")
- Drug intoxications (L-dopa, amphetamines; less commonly anticholinergics, antidepressants, lithium, phenytoin)*
- CNS complications of systemic metabolic disorders (e.g., hepatic or renal failure, hyperthyroidism, hypoparathyroidism, hypoglycemia, vasculitis)*
- Brain neoplasm (thalamic, basal ganglia)

NOTE. CNS = central nervous system. From Baldessarini et al. (1980).
* Both psychiatric disorder and dyskinesia may be present.

examinations: probable, withdrawal, transient, and persistent. Unfortunately, there are no clinical or laboratory tests that will establish a diagnosis of TD. Therefore, a process of differential diagnosis (largely by exclusion) remains essential.

Jeste and Wyatt (1982) have provided an excellent review of the diagnostic process in TD, and Granacher (1981) has also reviewed the differential diagnosis in detail.

A variety of techniques have been suggested for evaluating and rating TD once the diagnosis has been established; these have been most extensively reviewed by Gardos et al. (1977). In general, the methods involve electromechanical or imaging instrumentation, frequency counts, global ratings, or multiple-item ratings. These procedures have different advantages and disadvantages, and some combination of them is preferable when feasible.

EPIDEMIOLOGY

Prevalence

It is hoped that epidemiological studies will provide important clues to the risk factors and ultimately to the etiology and pathophysiology of TD. However, in this area, methodological differences and problems make the successful integration of available information somewhat difficult. Prevalence estimates may be influenced by the diagnostic criteria and assessment technique employed, patient characteristics (e.g., age and sex), the presence or absence of other neuromedical conditions, and treatment history characteristics (e.g., age at first treatment, length of neuroleptic exposure, etc.). In addition, the fact that administration of neuroleptics can mask the presence of TD also complicates prevalence estimates. It is not surprising, therefore, that the prevalence estimates have ranged from 0.5 to 57 percent. Kane and Smith (1982), in reviewing 56 studies, reported a mean (unweighted) prevalence of 20 percent among neuroleptic-treated samples. Jeste and Wyatt (1982) reviewing 37 studies (selected for minimum methodological requirements) found a weighted mean prevalence of 17.6 percent. It is likely that some proportion of these cases had movements that were not neuroleptic induced; nevertheless, it appears that abnormal involuntary movements are at least three times more prevalent in neuroleptic-treated patients as compared with patients unexposed to such drugs. It must be emphasized, however, that the drug-treated and non-drug-treated populations employed in making such comparisons are frequently not matched on important variables. The ideal study to assess the extent of the neuroleptic drug effect would involve random assignment to drug or placebo for a prolonged period of time— clearly not a practical design. The epidemiologic data, despite their limitations, provide compelling evidence that neuroleptic treatment is the single most important etiologic factor for involuntary movements in these patient populations.

Kane and Smith (1982) and Jeste and Wyatt (1981) found a substantial increase in the reported prevalence of TD over the last 20 years and concluded that despite numerous methodological problems, a true increase in prevalence probably has occurred.

The reported prevalence of SD in untreated populations has also varied widely (Kane and Smith 1982) with an unweighted mean of 5 percent. The highest rates have been reported in elderly, institutionalized patients, suggesting that age is an important factor. However, many individuals included in such surveys have suffered from a variety of neuromedical conditions, including various types of senile dementia, complicating any comparisons with neuroleptic-treated patients.

We have had the opportunity to examine two groups of healthy elderly volunteers in the community. The first series involved 127 individuals with an average age of 72 years, among whom 4 percent had abnormal involuntary movements (Kane et al. 1982a). In a second series, 400 individuals (average age of 73 years) were examined, yielding a prevalence of 1.2 percent (Lieberman et al. 1984).

Varga et al. (1982) reported a somewhat higher prevalence (10 percent) in a sample of 365 elderly individuals. A large proportion (236) of these subjects were patients in nursing homes. Medication histories were not available for individuals with no dyskinetic symptomatology; therefore, the denominator for the prevalence of SD in untreated individuals was only estimated. In addition, the large proportion of nursing home residents raises the possibility that neuromedical conditions that might play a role in the development of movement disorders were present in this population.

Klawans and Barr (1982) reported on 661 patients between the ages of 50 and 79 years without any history of neuroleptic exposure or known central nervous system disease and who were referred for neurologic evaluation not involving movement disorders (e.g., migraine, back pain, etc.). The prevalence of abnormal involuntary movements was 0.8 percent between 50 and 59 years of age, 6 percent between 60 and 69 years of age, and 7.8 percent between 70 and 79 years of age. It is difficult to tell, however, whether comparable "thresholds" for identifying a "case" of SD were used in these different investigations.

In general, data from these studies suggest that SDs do occur in the elderly, but not to a degree that could fully account for the high prevalence of presumptive TD observed in neuroleptic-treated elderly patients. Whether or not there is a higher proportion of false-positive TD diagnoses in elderly than in nonelderly drug-treated populations remains to be determined. These findings certainly underscore the importance of attempting a careful differential diagnosis and assessing to the extent possible the direct causal relationship between drug exposure and onset of movements. In addition, the importance of careful examination prior to initiation of neuroleptic treatment to determine the presence or absence of preexisting movement disorders cannot be emphasized enough.

The question as to whether schizophrenic illness itself may be responsible for abnormal movements is difficult to address now that the overwhelming majority of well-diagnosed schizophrenics have had some exposure to neuroleptics. Owens et al. (1982) reported on a group of chronically institutionalized schizophrenic patients who had apparently not received neuroleptics. A substantial proportion (53 percent) of these 47 individuals received positive ratings on scales to assess abnormal involuntary movements.

It should be noted that the average age of these patients was 67 years and the average length of institutionalization was 27 years.

We have not found any evidence of abnormal movements among 12 schizophrenic patients with no history of drug treatment or among 16 additional subjects with <1 month of total lifetime exposure. In addition, there are numerous reports in the literature of nonschizophrenic individuals, particularly those with affective illness, who have developed TD following, in some cases, relatively short courses of neuroleptics. Our own preliminary data from a prospective study suggest that patients with affective illness may be at a greater risk than schizophrenic persons for developing TD (Kane et al. 1983). Reports from other investigators have suggested a similar conclusion (Rosenbaum et al. 1977; Gardos et al. 1983).

Incidence

Few reports have focused on the prospective assessment of TD among psychiatric patients. Prevalence surveys provide useful information, but the limitations of retrospective data collection make the identification of possible risk factors difficult. In addition, point prevalence does not provide information on the duration or course of the movement disorder. For example, the prevalence of TD may be higher in the elderly because the condition is more persistent in that population (Smith and Baldessarini 1980), whereas the incidence may not be increased to the same extent.

We have reported preliminary results (Kane et al. 1982b, 1983, 1984) from an ongoing prospective study of TD development involving more than 800 psychiatric patients (mean age 27 years, median length of drug exposure at study entry 19 months). Patients were selected without consideration of diagnosis or drug treatment history. Approximately 10 percent of the entire sample has never received neuroleptics. These patients serve as a control group and allow us to keep the raters blind to treatment history. Patients are systematically reexamined every 3 months on rating scales to assess TD and drug-induced parkinsonism. A presumptive diagnosis of TD is made when three independent raters agree, after separate examinations, that the patient has at least mild TD based on a global judgment item included in a modified version of the Simpson Dyskinesia Scale. At that point the patient undergoes a battery of clinical laboratory tests and a neurological evaluation to rule out other possible causes of the movement disorder. An attempt is made to reduce or preferably discontinue neuroleptic drug treatment, and patients are followed biweekly whenever possible, with the hope that a longitudinal perspective will be useful in validating the diagnosis as well as in relating risk factors not only to incidence but also to outcome.

The results of a life table analysis involving the first 554 at-risk (i.e., neuroleptic-treated) subjects indicate that after 4 years of cumulative neuroleptic exposure, the incidence of TD is 14 percent (95 percent confidence interval 10–18 percent; see Figure 1). Using the categories included in the research diagnosis for TD (Schooler and Kane 1982), 47 percent of the cases that developed were considered persistent in that their symptoms continued for at least 3 months (either receiving or not receiving neuroleptics). Three months is a brief and somewhat arbitrary period, and longer

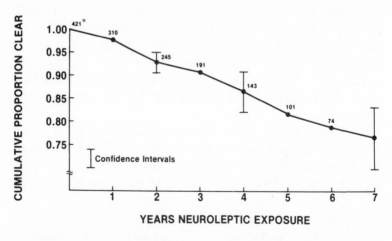

Figure 1   Tardive dyskinesia over 7 years of neuroleptic exposure. * Number of subjects entering each interval.

follow-up is necessary to characterize the ultimate course of the disorder. In addition, outcome will vary depending upon criteria used to define remission and duration of follow-up; e.g., a remission following drug discontinuation could be followed by a recurrence and subsequent persistence on return to neuroleptics.

Figure 2 presents the long-term outcome of TD in these patients, with "remission" defined according to three different

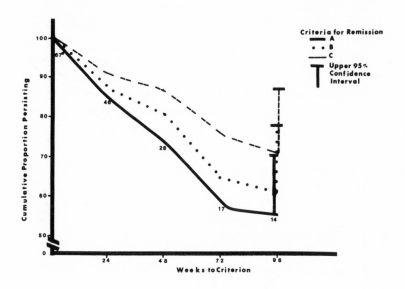

Figure 2 Tardive dyskinesia (TD) outcome. Criterion definition— A: Patient is rated as not having definite TD on at least two consecutive exams encompassing at least a 3-month period. (Ratings subsequent to this remission are ignored.) B: As in (A) above *plus* ratings subsequent to the 3-month remission may not exceed "questionable" on the global item for a continuous 3-month period (i.e., if remission is followed by a period of persistent TD, outcome is considered persistent). C: As in (A) above *plus* ratings subsequent to the 3-month remission may not exceed "questionable" on *any* exam (i.e., if remission is followed by any return of definite TD, outcome is considered persistent). * Number entering each interval.

criteria: TD remitted for a 3-month period (regardless of subsequent outcome); TD remitted for a 3-month period without a
subsequent recurrence that persists for 3 months; TD remitted and
no recurrence at all (at any single examination) throughout the
entire period of follow-up. Using the most stringent criterion at 96
weeks of follow-up, 75 percent of these patients had persistent
dyskinesia.

Figure 3 displays the outcome (using the first criterion above)
for those patients developing TD with fewer than 2 years of
cumulative neuroleptic exposure in contrast to those with longer
exposure. Outcome appears to be better for those with less
exposure; however, this variable is significantly correlated with
the likelihood of patients being withdrawn from neuroleptics
following TD development. As seen in Figure 4, this factor also
contributes to TD outcome, with those patients off drug for >50
percent of the follow-up interval being more likely to have a

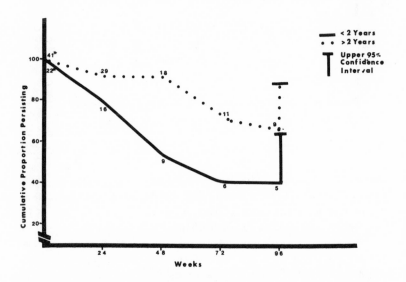

Figure 3 Tardive dyskinesia (TD) outcome by neuroleptic exposure
prior to TD development. Outcome criterion as in (A) for Figure
1. *Number entering each interval.

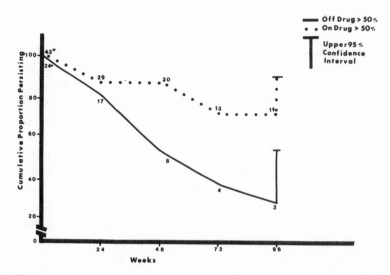

Figure 4 Tardive dyskinesia outcome by neuroleptic exposure during follow-up. Outcome criterion as in (A) for Figure 1. * Number entering each interval.

remission of TD. A larger number of patients will be necessary to attempt to statistically tease apart these factors.

It is also very important to note that among the patients developing TD in our sample, after an average length of follow-up of 30 months, 49 percent were never rated more than mild, 24 percent had more than one rating of moderate, and only 8 percent ever had a rating of moderately severe. This suggests that in this population, despite the continued presence of symptoms in many cases, there is little evidence of substantial progression or worsening of symptoms.

Recent reports from other investigators (Casey 1983a; Gardos et al. 1983) support this conclusion as well. There are patients, however, who do develop a very severe form of the disorder, and it has been our impression that many of these cases evolve very rapidly and may represent a distinct subtype. The intensive study of these patients may prove to be particularly revealing in terms of risk factors (Kane et al. 1980).

RISK FACTORS

It is apparent from epidemiologic reviews that the majority of neuroleptic-treated patients do not develop TD. In order to prevent the disorder from developing, the identification of those factors contributing to individual vulnerability would be very helpful. Numerous studies have suggested a variety of risk factors; however, in general, the data available in the literature are limited by important methodological problems, e.g., use of different criteria to make a diagnosis of TD, varying efforts to rule out false positives, retrospective data collection on treatment history variables, etc. In addition, it is difficult to find ideal controls, since patient groups that are similar on any one characteristic may differ significantly on other important variables.

Despite this, some important leads have been suggested. The single most frequently implicated risk factor is patient age. Dating the onset of TD, however, is difficult, making overestimation of age at TD onset somewhat likely. Despite this, the evidence seems quite strong that increasing age among neuroleptic-treated patients does increase the risk of developing TD as well as the severity and persistence of the condition.

Female sex is the second most frequently suggested risk factor. It does appear that women have a somewhat higher overall prevalence than men; however, samples of men and women were not always matched on other relevant variables (e.g., age). In addition, the ratio of women to men increases as the criterion used to define TD becomes more severe. Therefore, it appears that severer forms of the disorder are likely to develop in women. Whether sex differences in TD vulnerability reflect differences in other factors such as treatment history or underlying biological differences remains to be determined.

Drug type is an important issue both on clinical and heuristic grounds. At present, there are very few data to clearly implicate specific drugs or drug classes as increasing the risk of TD. There are enormous methodological problems in studying this issue. In order to establish relative risk, one would essentially have to assume some randomness in drug assignment as well as control for dosage and other relevant variables. In addition, given the enormous interindividual differences in drug absorption and metabolism, blood levels would be ideal in making comparisons, particularly in view of the possibility that blood levels following similar oral doses may be higher in patients with TD than in controls (Jeste et al. 1982). (The role of blood levels remains controversial, however, and further work is needed to clarify this issue.)

Cumulative drug exposure will be determined by both dosage and duration of administration. Given the epidemiologic evidence implicating neuroleptic drugs in the etiology of TD, it has generally been assumed that the risk of this disorder would increase with increasing cumulative exposure. As Kane and Smith (1982) have suggested, attempts at identifying dose-response curves for TD are made difficult by the relative infrequency of the condition (i.e., 15 percent corrected prevalence), the retrospective nature of most available data, and the methodological problems inherent in assessing pharmacologic variables. It is not surprising, therefore, that relatively few studies have been able to demonstrate a statistically significant relationship between increasing drug exposure and risk of TD. (This issue will be discussed further in the section on prevention).

Other risk factors that have been discussed in the literature include the presence of organic mental dysfunction, vulnerability to early clinically significant extrapyramidal side effects, prolonged use of anticholinergic medications, neuroleptic-free intervals, and diagnosis.

Data from our prospective study suggest that vulnerability to the development of early clinically significant extrapyramidal side effects may indicate vulnerability to subsequent development of TD, particularly for those patients who develop the disorder with relatively brief (<2 years) neuroleptic exposure.

We have also found that diagnosis does appear to be a risk factor. A life table analysis employing length of drug exposure and comparing the cumulative incidence of TD in patients with affective or schizoaffective disorder with that in patients diagnosed as schizophrenic suggests that the former have a significantly greater incidence of TD after 6 years of total neuroleptic exposure

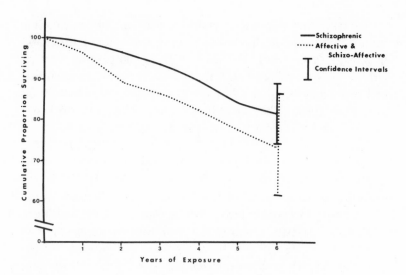

Figure 5   Tardive dyskinesia over 6 years of neuroleptic exposure by diagnosis.

(26 ± 13 percent for affective and schizoaffective compared with 18 ± 7 percent for schizophrenic patients; see Figure 5).

Evidence supporting these factors remains limited and again complicated by major methodological difficulties. See Jeste and Wyatt (1982) and Kane and Smith (1982) for reviews of risk factors.

ETIOLOGY

The evidence that implicates neuroleptic drugs in the etiology of TD is mainly epidemiologic, but very compelling. Despite this, the mechanism by which neuroleptic drugs lead to the development of this illness remains to be fully determined.

Several observations have suggested that TD may result from a state of relative dopaminergic hyperactivity. For example, the condition tends to become apparent or worsen upon withdrawal of neuroleptic medication. Given the putative mechanism of action of neuroleptics as the blockade of dopamine (DA) receptors, this serves to implicate the dopaminergic system. In addition, TD can resemble the dyskinesias produced by DA agonists or L-dopa in patients with Parkinson's disease. The administration of DA agonists or L-dopa has also been observed to exacerbate TD (though not consistently). The fact that this condition can be reduced or entirely suppressed by the administration of DA receptor blockers (neuroleptics) or DA-depleting agents (reserpine, tetrabenazine, α-methyl-p-tyrosine) provides additional evidence to support this hypothesis.

Anticholinergic drugs generally tend to either exacerbate or have little effect on TD, whereas in Parkinson's disease these drugs have a therapeutic effect. These observations taken together have suggested that the parkinsonian state and TD may reflect opposite ends of the same spectrum (Parkinson's disease resulting from a deficit of DA in nigrostriatal dopaminergic tracts as opposed to TD, which may be associated with nigrostriatal dopaminergic hyperactivity).

Numerous animal studies have been carried out that support the hypothesis of a postsynaptic DA receptor hypersensitivity occurring in animals following chronic neuroleptic treatment. Unfortunately, there is relatively little parallel evidence in humans.

Neuroleptic-treated monkeys have been reported to develop choreoathetosis and oral dyskinesias that in some cases persisted after cessation of treatment (Gunne and Barany 1976; Gunne 1983). These models may prove to be very useful in increasing our understanding of the disorder and could provide an opportunity to assess treatment strategies as well as to identify antipsychotic agents that might be free of this risk. See Jeste and Wyatt (1982) for a detailed review of biochemical hypotheses and animal models of TD.

TREATMENT

The literature on the treatment of TD has become vast and somewhat confusing. Many anecdotal and uncontrolled reports have encouraged the use of a specific treatment that was then found to be ineffective when subjected to a double-blind trial. In addition, differences in diagnostic criteria for and severity and duration of TD prior to institution of the experimental treatment have made comparisons across studies quite difficult. Jeste and Wyatt (1982) have reviewed in great detail treatment strategies for TD. They conclude that at present there is still no satisfactory treatment for most patients with the disorder.

Neuroleptics remain the most effective means of "suppressing" or "masking" the signs of TD; however, once the drug is withdrawn, the condition will recur. In addition, the fear remains that continued neuroleptic administration may ultimately exacerbate the disorder. Recent outcome studies, as discussed earlier, are encouraging, however, in suggesting that the majority of TD patients continued on neuroleptics for periods of up to 3 years do not experience any substantial increase of symptomatology while on the drugs (Kane et al. 1983; Gardos et al. 1983; Casey et al. 1983a). Withdrawal of neuroleptics remains the most desirable step, if clinically feasible, and remission of abnormal movements may occur in 30–40 percent of patients. The likelihood of improvement may decline with the increasing age of the patient and the increasing length of time neuroleptics are continued following the emergence of TD.

GABAergic drugs may have some effect in reducing signs of TD. Cholinergic agents may be useful in certain patients. In addition, it has been suggested that some patients benefit from a "down regulation" strategy involving administration and then withdrawal of DA agonists to reduce postsynaptic receptor hypersensitivity. The overall value of all of these treatments remains to be established.

PREVENTION

Until further knowledge is available concerning why some individuals are susceptible to TD and others are not, we are unable to offer definitive guidelines for prevention. Clearly, however, neuroleptics should be used only in those patients for whom no alternative treatment is available and for whom they have been shown to be of value. Neuroleptic drugs remain the mainstay of both acute and maintenance treatment for schizophrenia. An awareness of TD must enter into patient management. Prior to initiation of such drugs, patients should be examined to determine the presence of any preexisting movement disorders and they should be reexamined at periodic intervals. The lowest possible dose should be used for maintenance treatment. There are some prospective data suggesting that this strategy may have some impact on the incidence of TD (Kane et al. 1983).

If TD does develop, an attempt should be made to discontinue neuroleptics. The risk of relapse, however, is high in multiepisode schizophrenic patients withdrawn from neuroleptics for long periods of time. The best strategy for long-term neuroleptic treatment in patients who have developed TD has yet to be determined. Use of the lowest possible dose remains the major recommendation. Whether any particular drug or class of drugs offers an advantage in this situation remains hypothetical until appropriate controlled comparisons are made.

The patient and family should be involved in discussions about the benefits and risks of neuroleptic treatment from the outset, not just upon the emergence of TD. Clinicians should document in the chart the continued indications, continued benefit, attempts at dosage reduction, examinations for TD, as well as discussions with the patient and family regarding benefits and risks.

Despite the possibility of the development of TD, the benefits of neuroleptic treatment outweigh the risks in these circumstances. It is hoped that continued research will ultimately lead to safer drugs and/or more effective strategies for prevention.

References

Baldessarini RJ, Cole JO, Davis JM, et al: Tardive Dyskinesia: A Task Force Report of the American Psychiatric Association. Washington, DC, American Psychiatric Association, 1980

Casey DE: Tardive dyskinesia: what is the natural history? Int Drug Ther Newslett 18:13–16, 1983a

Casey, DE: Tardive dyskinesia and affective disorders. Paper presented at American Psychiatric Association, New York, NY, April 30–May 6, 1983b

Fann WE, Smith RC, Davis JM, et al., eds: Tardive Dyskinesia: Research and Treatment. New York, Spectrum Publications, 1980

Faurbye A, Rasch PJ, Petersen PB, et al: Neurological symptoms in pharmacotherapy of psychoses. Acta Psychiatr Scand 40:10–27, 1964

Gardos G, Cole JO, LaBrie R: The assessment of tardive dyskinesia. Arch Gen Psychiatry 34:1206–1212, 1977

Gardos G, Perenyi A, Cole JO: Tardive dyskinesia: changes after three years. J Clin Psychopharmacol 3:315–318, 1983

Granacher RP: Differential diagnosis of tardive dyskinesia: overview. Am J Psychiatry 138:1288–1297, 1981

Gualtieri CT, Bruening SE, Schroeder SR, et al: Tardive dyskinesia in mentally retarded children, adolescents, and young adults. Psychopharmacol Bull 18:62–65, 1982

Gunne LM: Studies on the pathophysiology of persistent neuroleptic-induced dyskinesia. Paper presented at American College of Neuropsychopharmacology, San Juan, Puerto Rico, December 1983

Gunne LM, Barany S: Haloperidol-induced tardive dyskinesia in monkeys. Psychopharmacology 50:237–340, 1976

Jeste DV, Wyatt RJ: Changing epidemiology of tardive dyskinesia. Am J Psychiatry 138:297–309, 1981

Jeste DV, Wyatt RJ: Understanding and Treating Tardive Dyskinesia. New York, Guilford Press, 1982

Jeste DV, Linnoila M, Wagner RL, et al: Serum neuroleptic concentrations and tardive dyskinesia. Psychopharmacology 76:377–380, 1982

Kane JM, Smith JM: Tardive dyskinesia: prevalence and risk factors, 1959–1979. Arch Gen Psychiatry 39:473–481, 1982

Kane JM, Struve FA, Weinhold B, et al: Strategy for the study of patients at high risk for tardive dyskinesia. Am J Psychiatry 137:1265–1267, 1980

Kane JM, Weinhold P, Kinon B, et al: Prevalence of abnormal involuntary movements ("spontaneous dyskinesias") in the normal elderly. Psychopharmacology 77:105–108, 1982a

Kane JM, Woerner M, Weinhold P, et al: A prospective study of tardive dyskinesia development: preliminary results. J Clin Psychopharmacol 2:345–349, 1982b

Kane JM, Rifkin A, Woerner M, et al: Low-dose neuroleptic treatment of outpatient schizophrenics. Arch Gen Psychiatry 40:893–896, 1983

Kane JM, Woerner M, Weinhold P, et al: Incidence of tardive dyskinesia: five year data from a prospective study. Psychopharmacol Bull 20:39–40, 1984

Klawans HL, Barr A: Prevalence of spontaneous lingual-facial-buccal dyskinesias in the elderly. Neurology 32:558–559, 1982

Lieberman J, Kane JM, Woerner M, et al: Prevalence of tardive dyskinesia in elderly samples. Psychopharmacol Bull 20:22–26, 1984

Owens DGC, Johnstone FC, Frith CD: Spontaneous involuntary disorders of movement. Arch Gen Psychiatry 39:452–461, 1982

Rosenbaum AH, Niven RG, Hansen NP, et al: Tardive dyskinesia: relationship with primary affective disorder. Dis Nerv Syst 38:423–427, 1977

Schonecker M: Ein eigentumliches Syndrom im oralen Bereich bei Megaphen Applikation. Nervenarzt 28:35, 1957

Schooler NR, Kane JM: Research diagnoses for tardive dyskinesia. Arch Gen Psychiatry 39:486–487, 1982

Sigwald J, Boutier D, Courvoisier S: Les accidents neurologiques des medications neuroleptiques. Rev Neurol (Paris) 100:553–595, 1959

Smith JM, Dunn DD: Sex differences in the prevalence of severe tardive dyskinesia. Am J Psychiatry 136:1080–1082, 1979

Smith JM, Baldessarini RJ: Changes in prevalence, severity and recovery in tardive dyskinesia with age. Arch Gen Psychiatry 37:1368–1373, 1980

Uhrbrand L, Faurbye A: Reversible and irreversible dyskinesia after treatment with perphenazine, chlorpromazine, reserpine and electroconvulsive therapy. Psychopharmacologia 1:408–418, 1960

Varga E, Sugarman AA, Varga V, et al: Prevalence of spontaneous oral dyskinesia in the elderly. Am J Psychiatry 139:329–331, 1982

6

Movement Disorders and Psychopathology

Dilip V. Jeste, M.D.
Craig N. Karson, M.D.
Richard Jed Wyatt, M.D.

6

Movement Disorders and Psychopathology

The association of movement disorders and psychopathology is of considerable interest to both clinicians and researchers. This chapter examines different aspects of that relationship. We will first review the literature on psychiatric disturbances in patients with spontaneously occurring movement disorders such as Huntington's disease (HD). We will then present data from our studies of psychopathology in patients with an iatrogenic movement disorder, tardive dyskinesia (TD).

SPONTANEOUS MOVEMENT DISORDERS AND PSYCHOPATHOLOGY

A number of investigators have reported a high incidence of psychiatric manifestations in HD, Parkinson's disease, and other movement disorders.

We wish to thank Theresa Hoffman for her expert secretarial assistance.

This chapter was written by the authors in their personal capacity, and does not necessarily reflect the views of the National Institute of Mental Health.

Studies in Individual Movement Disorders

HD. The association of HD with psychopathology has long been known. In his original report, George Huntington (1872) referred to "insanity with a tendency to suicide" as one of the hallmarks of the disorder. A number of psychiatric disturbances have since been described in HD patients. Table 1 enumerates the findings of major surveys of this disease published since 1960. There are some discrepancies in the results of different studies, which could be partly accounted for by differences in the methods used. Nevertheless there is a notable similarity in the overall findings (summarized in Table 2). Two-thirds of the patients manifested some form of psychopathology prior to the onset of chorea. The most common psychiatric diagnoses received by these patients during the "prodromal" period were neuroses (including anxiety states, neurasthenia, hysteria, neurotic depression) and

Table 1 Psychiatric Syndromes in Huntington's Disease: Individual Studies

	Prodromal		Presenting Signs	
	Oliver (1970)	Dewhurst et al. (1970)	Brothers (1964)	Heathfield (1967)
Total *N*	115	102	237	80
% Psychiatric Diagnosis	72	57	41	49
% Schizophrenia-like Psychoses	10	1	—	6
% Affective Disorders	30	7	—	6
Depression	At least 8	7	—	6
Mania	0	0	—	0
% Neuroses and Personality Disorders	At least 28	43	—	21
% Dementia	13	6	—	8
% Other Psychiatric Syndromes	?	0	—	4
% No Psychiatric Diagnosis	18	10	59	51
% Insufficient Data	0	33	—	0

Table 1 *(cont.)*

	Presenting Signs			
	James et al. (1969)	Bolt (1970)	Dewhurst et al. (1970)	Lieberman et al. (1979)
Total N	33	68	102	45
% Psychiatric Diagnosis	55	47	45	38
% Schizophrenia-like Psychoses	12	—	7	—
% Affective Disorders	3	—	9	—
Depression	3	—	—	—
Mania	0	—	—	—
% Neuroses and Personality Disorders	39	—	22	—
% Dementia	?	—	8	—
% Other Psychiatric Disorders	0	—	0	—
% No Psychiatric Diagnosis	45	53	55	62
% Insufficient Data	0	0	0	0

	Prevalence				
	Chandler et al. (1960)	Brothers (1964)	Heathfield (1967)	Bolt (1970)	Lieberman et al. (1979)
Total N	417	?	82	334	50
% Psychiatric Diagnosis	89	(155 admitted to mental hospital)	95	?	90
% Schizophrenia-like Psychoses	—	13	11	33	18
% Affective Disorders	—	11	?	?	38
Depression	—	9	12	25	38
Mania	—	2	5	?	0
% Neuroses and Personality Disorders	—	0	4	8	16
% Dementia	—	70	95	70	90
% Other Psychiatric Syndromes	—	10	11	?	—
% No Psychiatric Diagnosis	11	?	5	?	10
% Insufficient Data	0	?	—	—	0

Table 1 *(cont.)*

	Prevalence	
	Folstein et al. (1979)	Caine and Shoulson (1983)
Total *N*	11	30
% Psychiatric Diagnosis	100	80
% Schizophrenia-like Psychoses	18	10
% Affective Disorders	46	?
Depression	27	17
Mania	18	—
% Neuroses and Personality Disorders	36	50
		(including 6 dysthymics)
% Dementia	100	?*
% Other Psychiatric Syndromes	0	17
		(including 2 atypical psychoses and 1 paranoid psychosis)
% No Psychiatric Diagnosis	0	20
% Insufficient Data	0	0

NOTE. Some patients had more than one psychiatric diagnosis. Prodromal = prior to onset of chorea; presenting signs = signs (psychiatric) at the time of first hospitalization or first diagnosis of Huntington's disease; prevalence = prevalence (of psychiatric syndromes) in patients with diagnosed Huntington's disease having psychiatric follow-ups.

*Some degree of cognitive impairment was present in every patient.

Table 2 Huntington's Disease and Psychiatric Syndromes: A Summary

% Patients with	Prodromal*	Reason for First Admission†	Overall Prevalence‡
Psychiatric Diagnosis	65	46	91
Schizophrenia-like Psychosis	6	8	18
Affective Disorders	19	6	42
Neuroses and Personality Disorders	36	27	23
Dementia	10	8	89
Other	?	1	9

NOTE. Some patients had more than one psychiatric diagnosis. Based on studies by:
* Oliver (1970) and Dewhurst et al. (1970)
†Heathfield (1967), James et al. (1969), and Dewhurst et al. (1970)
‡Heathfield (1967), Bolt (1970), Lieberman et al. (1979), Folstein et al. (1979), and Caine and Shoulson (1983).

personality disorders (frequently described as "emotional instability"). In almost one-half of all patients, the reason for first hospitalization was psychiatric. Again, the diagnosis in a majority of these patients was neurosis or personality disorder. A psychiatric follow-up of the patients with diagnosed HD showed that over 90 percent had recognizable psychopathology. Some degree of dementia was present in almost all of these patients. (The characteristics of the dementia are discussed under Subcortical Dementia below.) Among the remaining psychiatric disturbances, affective disorders ranked highest (42 percent), with depression being much more prevalent than mania. An apparent reduction in the proportion of patients with neuroses and personality disorders at this stage (23 percent) may reflect the fact that some of the patients who receive such a diagnosis in the early stages of HD later go on to develop florid psychotic breakdowns. Eighteen percent of patients had a schizophreniform psychosis. These data do not support any definitive association between HD and specific psychiatric disorders. Also, the conventional psychiatric diagnoses may not provide the best framework for categorizing psychopathologic disturbances in HD. Whittier (1977) suggests that certain affect-related symptoms in HD patients, such as aggression and irritability, may be striatal release symptoms.

Several investigators have conducted neuropsychological testing in patients with HD. Lyle and Gottesman (1977) found that mild dementia might occur years before the disorder is diagnosed with certainty. Studies by Fedio et al. (1979) and Wexler (1979) suggest disorders of cognition, especially in the perceptual area, in HD patients and in those at risk for the disease. Wexler (1979) asks the provocative question of "whether these psychological deficits arise as a consequence of cortical destruction or whether the basal ganglia play some as yet unappreciated role in cognitive and emotional functioning." Norton (1975) and Fedio et al. (1979) reported that HD patients had abnormally high scores on the Minnesota Multiphasic Personality Inventory (MMPI) scales of depression, schizophrenia, and psychasthenia, although there could be some concern about the validity of these scales in demented patients.

Parkinson's Disease.   In his original description of the disease named after him, James Parkinson (1817) alluded to psychiatric manifestations such as depression and a terminal delirium. He and many subsequent investigators believed, however, that there was no dementia in Parkinson's disease. Yet, in the last few years, researchers have been impressed with a rather high incidence of dementia in this disorder (Table 3). Recent studies have noted that 30–80 percent of patients with Parkinson's disease have some degree of intellectual impairment [see the review by Mayeux and Stern (1983)]. Lieberman et al. (1979) noted that dementia occurred 10 times more often in parkinsonian patients than in their spouses and in age-matched normal controls from the literature. Bowen (1976) studied nearly 500 patients with Parkinson's disease and 200 normal controls on a variety of neuropsychological tests. She found that Parkinson's disease produced abnormalities in short-

Table 3   Psychiatric Syndromes in Movement Disorders

Movement Disorder	Psychiatric Syndrome	Prevalence	Comments
Parkinson's Disease	Dementia	50–60%	Possibly two types—Alzheimer's and the so-called "subcortical"
	Depression	40–50% (in nondemented patients)	Much higher in demented patients; difficulty in assessing depression
Tourette's Syndrome	Obsessive Compulsive Disorder	60–70%	Commoner in older patients and those with a family history of Tourette's
	Others	—	Include depression, schizophrenia, etc.
Sydenham's Chorea	Neurotic or Personality Disorders	70–75%	Possible association with schizophrenia
Meige's Syndrome	Depression	25–35%	—
Wilson's Disease	Dementia	About 50%	Associated with CT evidence of basal ganglia lesions
	Others	?	Affective disorders, etc.

NOTE.   CT = computed tomography.

term memory and concept formation similar to those found after penetrating trauma to the convexity of frontal lobes. There was, however, no primary sensory deficit. Boller et al. (1980), Sroka et al. (1981), and others have reported that parkinsonian patients with severe dementia or permanent organic mental syndrome tend to have clinical, radiographic, and neuropathologic changes similar to those seen in Alzheimer's disease. It is likely that there are two types of dementia in Parkinson's disease: Alzheimer type and the so-called "subcortical" type (discussed later).

A number of investigators have reported a high incidence of depression in Parkinson's disease. Lieberman et al. (1979) found depression in 38 of their 42 demented patients with Parkinson's disease. Mayeux et al. (1981) studied 55 patients with Parkinson's disease but without dementia. Using the Beck Depression Inventory, 47 percent were found to be depressed. Whether the depression in Parkinson's patients validly meets criteria for psychiatric diagnosis such as in the third edition of the Diagnostic and Statistical Manual of Mental Disorders (DSM-III; American Psychiatric Association 1980) is, however, unclear. As Parkinson's disease itself is characterized by signs such as psychomotor retardation, precise assessment of a depressive syndrome may be difficult.

Tourette's Syndrome. The presence of psychopathology in Tourette's syndrome (TS) has been well known ever since (and including) the original description by Gilles de la Tourette (1885). A variety of psychiatric disturbances including obsessive compulsive disorder, schizophrenia, alcoholism, depression, antisocial behavior, and hysterical personality disorder have been reported in TS patients (see Montgomery et al. 1982). Recent studies by Nee et al. (1980) and Montgomery et al. (1982) found a high prevalence (68 and 66 percent, respectively) of obsessive compulsive illness in patients with TS. The presence and severity of the compulsive behavior seemed to be positively related to the older age of the patients and to a positive family history of the syndrome.

Sydenham's Chorea (Chorea Minor). Sydenham's chorea is characterized by a sudden onset of irregular movements of a choreiform type in young patients. The chorea is regarded as a delayed manifestation of rheumatic fever, although "pure" chorea can be found in the absence of rheumatic signs (Stollerman 1983). A wide range of neuropathological changes have been described, including "rheumatic" changes in the cerebral vessels (Bruetsch 1940, 1944), inflammatory and degenerative changes (Grinber and Sahs 1966), and edema, congestion, and degeneration of neurons (Brain and Walton 1969). Because it is an encephalopathy, as in late HD, the evaluation of psychopathological features in patients with Sydenham's chorea becomes difficult. In a review of 175 cases, Schwartzman (1950) found that the most common psychiatric features were shyness, introversion, and a tendency to cry easily. Freeman et al. (1965) interviewed 40 patients 30 years after their acute illness and found that 33 of them suffered from either a personality disorder or a psychoneurosis compared with only 25 percent of the controls.

Perhaps more interesting is the suggested association between Syndenham's chorea and schizophrenia. Guttman (1936) first noted that a history of chorea was twice as common in schizophrenia as in manic-depressive illness. Soon afterward, Bruetsch (1940, 1944) performed autopsies on 100 consecutive schizophrenic patients and found that 9 percent had rheumatic valvular lesions of the heart. He also found that a small group of schizophrenic patients demonstrated cerebral endarteritis at autopsy, though to our knowledge this has not been confirmed in other studies.

A notable characteristic of Guttman's and Bruetsch's studies is that they did not rely primarily on clinical evaluations. Of interest is a recent retrospective study of 32 patients with Sydenham's chorea (Nausieda et al. 1983) in which it was found that one-half of the patients had received dopamine (DA) agonists and that some of them had had adverse reactions, either neurologic or psychiatric. These patients reporting adverse reactions had a significant elevation in their scores on the MMPI psychotic tetrad. Insofar as schizophrenia may also involve increased cerebral DA activity, this evidence is consistent with an association between chorea minor and schizophrenia.

Meige's Syndrome.   Meige's syndrome, a focal dystonia, involves blepharospasm and dystonias of the jaw. Its onset is usually in the fifth or sixth decade of life, and while not life threatening, Meige's syndrome can be extremely disabling. In a recent study that reawakened interest in this disorder, Mardsen (1976) noted that 14 of 39 patients with Meige's syndrome were depressed either before or at its onset. Tolosa (1981) confirmed this observation in 7 of 17 patients and found that depression antedated the movement disorder by <1 year in 5 of these 7 patients. One-fourth of the patients of Jankovic and Ford (1983) had depression before, at, or after the expression of their facial dystonia. Since the method of diagnosis of depression in these studies was retrospective and did not employ specific psychiatric diagnostic criteria, the interpretation of these findings is limited. Nevertheless, the replication of this association in three consecutive studies warrants future rigorous evaluation of psychopathology in Meige's syndrome.

Wilson's Disease.   In his classic description of hepatolenticular degeneration, S. A. Kinner Wilson (1912) stressed the association of hepatic cirrhosis with tremor, rigidity, dysarthria, dysphagia, and emotional disturbances. Wilson's disease, transmitted as an autosomal recessive trait, is associated with a deficiency of the copper-binding serum enzyme ceruloplasmin. Copper is deposited in various tissues. Clinical manifestations include jaundice, Kayser-Fleischer ring in the cornea, "wing-beating" tremor, and a variety of psychiatric syndromes. Dobyns et al. (1979) found that psychiatric disorders occurred in 19 of 44 patients with Wilson's disease who had neurologic symptoms. In five of these patients, "significant psychiatric syndromes of recent onset" were present at the time of clinical onset of the disease. Pandey et al. (1981) described a patient with Wilson's disease whose manic symptoms improved on treatment with fusaric acid, an inhibitor of dopamine-β-hydroxylase. Kendall et al. (1981) studied computed tomography (CT) scans of 12 patients with Wilson's disease. Seven of the patients had signs of intellectual deterioration. All of these seven patients had CT evidence of either low density or atrophy of basal ganglia. There was only a moderate correlation between cerebral atrophy and the degree of dementia.

Methodological Issues

Before discussing possible interpretations of above-mentioned literature, we must first consider the various methodological issues involved in those studies.

Design of Study.   Retrospective studies relying on the descriptions given in patient charts are obviously less satisfactory (although easier to complete) than long-term prospective investigations. The use of control groups (both with other types of movement disorders and without any movement disorder) is highly recommended. Unfortunately, a majority of studies of psychiatric disturbances in patients with movement disorders have been retrospective and uncontrolled.

Patient Selection.   The prevalence of psychopathology would be high if only the patients referred to a psychiatric department were selected. Brothers (1964) reported on psychiatric disorders in 155 patients with HD admitted to a mental hospital. His findings are not likely to be generalizable to HD patients at large. In contrast, Folstein et al. (1979) studied HD patients referred to the genetics clinic or neurology department.

Patient Characteristics.   Variables such as age, gender, socioeconomic status, and educational level may affect the prevalence and intensity of neuropsychiatric syndromes. In Parkinson's disease, for example, intellectual impairment has been reported to be related to age at onset of the disease (Lieberman et al. 1979).

Diagnosis of Movement Disorders.   In the final analysis, the diagnosis of most movement disorders is based on clinical judgment. Diagnostic reliability and validity can be increased by using a set of standard diagnostic criteria. This is especially true for conditions such as TS that have a wide quantitative and qualitative spectrum of clinical manifestations (see Chapter 2).

Disease Characteristics.   Psychopathology may be related to the severity of the movement disorder, the stage of the illness, the type of symptoms, etc. Thus, the prevalence of various neuropsychiatric syndromes is somewhat different at different phases of HD (Table 2).

Sroka et al. (1981) reported that organic mental syndrome was diagnosed 4.5 times more often in "atypical" parkinsonian patients than in "typical" ones. "Atypical" parkinsonism was defined as an extrapyramidal dysfunction of a parkinsonian nature, accompanied by evidence of the involvement of other system(s) such as the pyramidal tract, cerebellum, etc.

Assessment of psychopathology.   Recent studies have used standard diagnostic criteria for psychiatric illnesses [e.g., DSM-III criteria in the study by Caine and Shoulson (1983)]. It is, of course, debatable whether disorders such as depression occurring in patients with organic mental syndrome are pathophysiologically identical to those occurring in patients without brain damage. This issue cannot be settled satisfactorily at present. Approximate quantification of the psychopathology is also important. Hence, the use of standardized psychiatric rating scales is preferred, although many scales have their own limitations in terms of reliability and validity.

Interpretation of Observed Association Between Movement Disorder and Psychopathology

A number of possible explanations, neither mutually exclusive nor jointly exhaustive, should be considered in interpreting an observed association between a given movement disorder and certain kinds of psychopathology. As an example, we will consider probable explanations for the reported association between HD and depression (Table 2) (also see Chapter 3).

Coincidental Association.   Depression occurs in a certain percentage of the general population. The prevalence of depression in HD is, however, considerably greater than what could be explained on the basis of chance alone.

Reactive Depression.   Persons with debilitating and fatal disorders such as HD are obviously prone to become depressed. The depression in HD patients is not always reactive, however, as the onset of depression precedes the appearance of chorea and the diagnosis of the disease in a sizable proportion of patients (Table 1).

Iatrogenic Depression.   Certain drugs used in the treatment of HD (including neuroleptics) may cause signs of depression. This is again an unlikely explanation for the depression that precedes the diagnosis and treatment of the disease.

Genetic Linkage.   The genes for depression and HD could be closely linked. The available data do not allow us to either confirm or refute this hypothesis.

Neurochemical Similarity.   The presence of generalized disturbance in the activity of certain neurotransmitters could explain both the movement disorder and the psychopathology. It is thus logical that Parkinson's disease is frequently associated with depression, since reduced catecholaminergic activity is believed to underlie both the conditions. On the other hand, there is *relative* dopaminergic overactivity in HD (Marsden 1982). Hence, the association of HD and depression may be difficult to explain on the basis of decreased catecholaminergic activity. Such a hypothesis cannot yet be dismissed, however, because our knowledge of the neurochemical pathology in these disorders is still very inadequate. Also, "catecholaminergic activity" is too broad a term. The ever-increasing data on the various subpopulations of DA and norepinephrine receptors indicate that there is a risk of oversimplification if we rely on the neurochemical concepts of a decade ago.

Cerebral Cortical Damage.   In HD, atrophic changes are not restricted to the striatum, but also involve certain other regions including the frontal cortex. Lesions of the frontal cortex can help explain the associated depression. Yet, there is no consistent relationship between cortical atrophy and depression in HD. Indeed, even the dementia seen in HD, Wilson's disease, Parkinson's disease, and other movement disorders does not often correlate highly with the extent of cortical atrophy present on the CT scan. Clinically, too, typical signs of cortical involvement such as aphasia, alexia, apraxia, and agonsia are absent in demented or depressed patients with HD (and sometimes Parkinson's disease).

Subcortical Dementia. Several groups of investigators have proposed that the characteristic behavioral changes seen in patients with HD (McHugh, unpublished data; cited by Mayeux et al. 1983), progressive supranuclear palsy (Albert et al. 1974), Parkinson's disease (Albert 1978; Marsden 1978), and Wilson's disease (Benson 1983) are different from those found in patients with Alzheimer-type "cortical" dementia. The dementia in the patients with primary movement disorders (having predominantly basal ganglionic lesions) has sometimes been termed "subcortical" dementia.

Clinical characteristics of the putative subcortical dementia (Benson 1983) include: abnormal involuntary movements; psychomotor retardation; forgetfulness without inability to learn new material; situation-dependent apathy; and the absence of cortical signs such as aphasia or apraxia. In contrast to the Alzheimer-type dementia, there is a notable improvement in psychomotor retardation, forgetfulness, and apathy with support, reassurance, and encouragement.

The concept of subcortical dementia has been criticized (Victor 1978) on the grounds that the conditions included under that term (e.g., HD, Parkinson's disease) are associated with cortical atrophy too. Also, recent work showing a degeneration of the subcortical cholinergic neurons in the nucleus basalis of Meynert (Whitehouse et al. 1982) indicates that Alzheimer's dementia too may involve subcortical structures. Recently Mayeux et al. (1983) compared the neuropsychological performance of patients with Alzheimer's disease, Parkinson's disease, and HD and concluded that the pattern of neuropsychologic impairment in the three groups was not distinct. There were several methodological and conceptual problems with this study: The only instrument used for neuropsychological testing was the Mini-Mental State Examination rather than a test battery such as Luria's; different scales for functional disability were employed for the three groups; and there was a marked difference in the numbers of patients (e.g., among those with Mini-Mental State scores of 30–20, the authors compared 1 patient with HD, 3 with Parkinson's disease, and 14 with Alzheimer's disease using parametric statistics). In fact, some of the data clearly suggest a difference between Alzheimer's and Huntington's dementias. (As we mentioned earlier, Parkinson's dementia may include both types.) The degree of dementia was much milder even in late-stage HD patients as compared with Alzheimer's. Depression was notably more common in HD and parkinsonian patients.

We believe that there is some value to the concept of clinically different subtypes of dementia with somewhat different neuropathologic bases. The terms "cortical" and "subcortical" dementias may, however, be overly simplistic. This unfortunate choice of words may have blurred the utility of distinguishing between at least two possible, albeit overlapping, subcategories of dementia. Here a question arises: Can lesions of subcortical structures produce dementia? To put it in another way: Are subcortical structures such as basal ganglia concerned with higher mental functions to any significant extent?

Basal Ganglia and Higher Mental Functions

Traditionally, the so-called higher mental functions such as intellect, memory, and language have been believed to depend primarily on the cerebral cortex. Yet, there is a growing body of evidence to indicate that certain subcortical structures such as basal ganglia may also contribute to such higher functions. Some of those considerations will be outlined here. [There are also data linking lesions of other subcortical structures such as thalamus to dementia (see Wallesch et al. 1983). We will not review those data, however, since lesions of structures beside the basal ganglia are not thought to be primarily responsible for the movement disorders described in this chapter.]

Basal ganglia consist of subcortical gray masses derived predominantly from the telencephalon. The terms "basal ganglia," "extrapyramidal system," and "nigrostriatal system" are often used interchangeably (and erroneously). Basal ganglia include the corpus striatum (comprising the caudate, putamen, and globus pallidus) and, according to some authors, the substantia nigra, subthalamic nucleus of Luys, claustrum, and amygdaloid nuclear complex (Carpenter 1976; Adams and Victor 1981). These nuclear masses are believed to be concerned with the control of the motor system.

Developmental Considerations. Both the cerebral cortex and most of the basal ganglia are embryologically derived from the same structure, i.e., the telencephalon. (The subthalamic nucleus of Luys is derived from the diencephalon and the pars compacta of the substantia nigra from the mesencephalon.) Phylogenetically, basal ganglia are older than the cerebral cortex. In animals without a cortex or with a poorly developed one, the corpus striatum is the most important forebrain center; along with the diencephalon, it constitutes the highest sensorimotor integrating mechanism (Carpenter 1976).

Fiber Connections. The striatum receives input from all the major sensory, suprasensory (multimodal), and limbic areas of the cerebral cortex. The entire neocortex projects to the striatum (Graybiel and Ragsdale 1979). Striatal output is directed primarily through the pallidum (and substantia nigra) to the "motor thalamus" and thence to the premotor, rolandic, and somatosensory areas of the cortex. Striatal afferents from and efferents to the cerebral cortex and thalamus are topographically organized. There is thus a closed feedback loop between the striatum and the cerebral cortex. The striatum is not merely a motor structure that mediates a collateral aspect of the generation of movement (DaMasio et al. 1982); rather, it is a principal programmer of "movement" (in a broad sense of that term) in relation to ongoing multimodal perception and imagery, and, in all probability, also plays a role in the organization of perception (Teuber 1976).

Aphasia with Lesions of Basal Ganglia.   DaMasio et al. (1982) and Naeser et al. (1982) have described atypical aphasias in patients with nonhemorrhagic infarcts in the striatum on the dominant side. (There were no suspect cortical areas on the CT scans.) Similar lesions in the nondominant hemisphere were not associated with aphasia. Naeser et al. (1982) reported that nearly 10 percent of the aphasia cases on their file during the previous 2 years had striatal lesions on the CT scans.

Binswanger's Disease (Chronic Progressive Subcortical Encephalopathy).   Although this is a controversial entity, a number of cases of presumed Binswanger's disease have been described in the literature (e.g., DeReuck et al. 1980; Loizou et al. 1981). Characteristic features include acute and subacute neurologic deficits with dementia in hypertensive or arteriosclerotic patients. CT scans show white matter low attenuation with predominantly subcortical infarcts. Postmortem examination of the brain reveals demyelination, cerebral arteriosclerosis, infarcts in basal ganglia and thalami, and ventricular dilatation, with preservation of cerebral cortex.

Possible Relationship to Schizophrenia.   Lidsky et al. (1979) have discussed the possible role of basal ganglia dysfunction in schizophrenia. Bowman and Lewis (1980) enumerated sites of subcortical pathology in 22 neurological disorders clinically resembling schizophrenia, and reported that the basal ganglia were the most commonly involved structures in these conditions.

Animal Studies.   Teuber's review of the literature (1976) concludes that in all the species studied, lesions of basal ganglia produce more than purely motor difficulties; they also cause characteristic perceptual and cognitive deficits. The behavioral alterations seen following basal ganglia lesions parallel, in several respects, the known effects of selective cortical ablations. In the very young, some of the functions of the basal ganglia might substitute for the as-yet-undeveloped functions of the cortex.

In summary, there is evidence from several different sources that seems to suggest that the basal ganglia may be partially involved in the regulation of higher mental functions. The nature or extent of such involvement is, however, entirely unclear at the present time. Stern (1983) has reviewed data indicating that the basal ganglia form an important part of a feedback system that regulates perceptual motor coordination by correlating and integrating motor and sensory information. Lesions in specific parts of the basal ganglia could therefore produce disturbances of higher-order control of movement, manifesting in impairment of certain behavioral and intellectual tasks and presenting as abnormal movements and some types of psychopathology. It is conceivable that subcortical lesions produce certain disturbances of mental status by interfering with pathways leading to the frontal cortex. There is an ongoing interaction between cortical and subcortical structures. Most dementias probably involve disturbances of both, although the relative proportions would vary. In certain dementias associated with movement disorders, lesions of the basal ganglia may be predominantly responsible for some types of impairments in higher mental functions.

IATROGENIC MOVEMENT DISORDERS AND PSYCHOPATHOLOGY

Literature Review

There have been relatively few systematic studies of the relationship between iatrogenic movement disorders and psychopathology. The most common such disorders are due to extrapyramidal side effects of neuroleptics. Neuroleptics are prescribed primarily for the treatment of psychotic disorders. The efficacy of these drugs in controlling different psychiatric symptoms is variable. Also, there is no consistent relationship between therapeutic effects and side effects of neuroleptics. These considerations point to difficulties in interpreting observed associations between neuroleptic-induced movement disorders and specific psychopathology.

The most serious movement disorder commonly produced by neuroleptics is TD (Jeste and Wyatt 1981). Several groups of investigators have reported a somewhat increased prevalence of TD in patients with major affective disorders, especially depression (see Chapter 5). It is, however, uncertain whether this increased prevalence is due to a direct relationship between dyskinesia and depression, or to certain treatment-related variables such as intermittent neuroleptic use in patients with affective disorders (see Jeste and Wyatt, 1982b). Cutler et al. (1981) noted that the severity of dyskinesia in two of their bipolar patients correlated positively with the intensity of depression, whereas Keshavan and Goswamy (1982) found just the opposite in a patient whose dyskinesia became worse during manic episodes. Glazer et al. (1984) observed an inverse correlation between the intensity of depression and that of dyskinesia in their schizophrenic patients.

Degkwitz (1969) and Hippius and Lange (1970) reported a positive correlation between the severity of psychosis and that of dyskinesia. Hamra et al. (1983) noticed a higher prevalence of TD in patients with paranoid schizophrenia. Chouinard and Jones (1980) proposed that some dyskinetic patients have a so-called "supersensitivity psychosis" characterized predominantly by positive symptoms of schizophrenia. They attributed this to the supersensitivity of mesolimbic DA receptors. It is, however, unclear whether the postulated neurochemical basis is valid.

In summary, there is a heterogeneity of findings in the published literature on a relationship between TD and specific psychopathology. Below we will describe two studies that we recently carried out to address this issue (Jeste et al. 1984; Karson et al., unpublished data).

Recent Studies

Forty-seven patients who were admitted to the research wards of the National Institute of Mental Health and who met the research

diagnostic criteria for schizophrenia (Spitzer et al. 1977) were
included in the study. At least two trained nurses rated the
patients "blind" (with respect to medication) twice a day using the
Brief Psychiatric Rating Scale (BPRS; Overall and Gorham 1962).
In addition, the patients were rated biweekly on the Abnormal
Involuntary Movement Scale (AIMS; National Institute of Mental
Health 1975), the abbreviated version of Simpson's Rockland
Tardive Dyskinesia Rating Scale (Simpson et al. 1979), and the
Simpson-Angus Extra-Pyramidal Side Effect Rating Scale (Simpson
and Angus 1970).

Seventeen of the 47 patients were diagnosed as having TD on
the basis of specific criteria (Table 4). Each of these TD patients
had a mean AIMS global rating of at least two on the zero to four

Table 4 Research Criteria for Tardive Dyskinesia

(A) Phenomenology
   1) Choreoathetoid or rhythmic abnormal involuntary movements, reduced by
      voluntary movements of affected body parts and increased by those of
      unaffected areas, and absent during sleep
   2) Involvement of one or more of these areas: tongue, jaw, and extremities

(B) Onset and Duration
   1) Onset after at least 3 months of neuroleptic treatment; appearance of dyskinesia
      either during a course of drug treatment or within a few weeks of neuroleptic
      withdrawal
   2) Duration: At least 3 weeks

(C) Pharmacologic Response
   1) Temporary suppression by increasing neuroleptic dose, and aggravation by dose
      reduction or discontinuation
   2) Nonresponse to or aggravation by anticholinergic drugs (possible exception:
      certain tardive dystonias)

(D) Differential Diagnosis
   1) Exclude tremors, acute dystonias, myoclonus, mannerisms, and compulsions
   2) Rule out other causes of dyskinesia such as Huntington's disease, Wilson's
      disease, ill-fitting dentures, etc.

(E) Severity
   1) Mean global rating of at least 2 on the zero to four Abnormal Involuntary
      Movement Scale

NOTE. Modified from Jeste and Wyatt (1982b).

scale. At the end of the study, TD patients were divided into persistent versus intermittent TD groups. In persistent TD patients ($N = 8$), the AIMS global rating remained at two or higher throughout their hospital stay (mean six months). Those TD patients ($N = 9$) whose AIMS global score fell to one or zero on at least two successive biweekly assessments were designated as having intermittent TD.

Study 1. All 47 patients were withdrawn from psychotropic medications for a period of at least 4 weeks. The mean BPRS ratings during the last 2 weeks were taken as an index of the neuroleptic-free psychopathology of these patients. The mean BPRS scores (total as well as individual syndrome subscales) for the three groups of patients (persistent TD, intermittent TD, and non-TD) were compared.

The three patient groups were similar in terms of age, gender

Table 5 A Comparison of the Three Patient Groups (Study 1)

	Persistent TD ($N = 8$)	Intermittent TD ($N = 9$)	Non-TD ($N = 30$)
Age (years)	35 ± 6	34 ± 7	30 ± 8
Gender (M/F)	3/5	6/3	20/10
Duration of Illness (years)	14 ± 7	11 ± 5	11 ± 5

NOTE. Values (except for gender) represent means $\pm$ SD. TD = tardive dyskinesia.

Table 6 Brief Psychiatric Rating Scale Syndrome Scores: Number of Patients with Scores Above Median Values (Study 1)

	Persistent TD ($N = 8$)	Intermittent TD ($N = 9$)	Non-TD ($N = 30$)
Depression	7	5	12**
Anxiety	1	4	19*
Negative Symptoms	5	7	12**

NOTE. TD = tardive dyskinesia.
* $p < .05$, Fisher's exact probability test.
** $p < .07$.

distribution, and duration of schizophrenia (Table 5). There were no significant differences on any of the six BPRS syndrome scores (depression, positive symptoms, negative symptoms, paranoia, anxiety, and activation) between the TD and non-TD patients (Mann-Whitney U test; Seigel 1956).

Significant differences or trends were found, however, when examining the proportionality of patients about the median scores on the BPRS subscales (Table 6). A significantly lower proportion of TD patients (5 of 17) had anxiety syndrome scores (comprised of tension and anxiety statement items) above the overall median value as compared with nondyskinetic patients (19 of 30; $p < .04$, Fisher's exact probability test). This was particularly clear in patients with persistent dyskinesia, as only one of eight had a score above the median ($p < .05$). Twelve of the 17 patients with TD had a depression score (comprised of guilt feelings, depressed mood, helplessness/hopelessness, and somatic concern items) equal to or greater than the median depression score for all patients. This was true in only 12 of 30 nondyskinetic patients ($p < .07$). Within the group with TD, seven of eight patients with persistent dyskinesia had a depression score equal to or above the median ($p < .05$) compared with five of nine patients with intermittent dyskinesia ($p < .4$). There was a similar trend for patients with TD: A higher percentage (12 of 17) had negative symptom scores (comprised of emotional withdrawal, motor retardation, and blunted affect items) above the median score compared with nondyskinetic patients (12 of 30; $p < .07$).

Depression scores in all the patients correlated significantly with those of withdrawal ($r_s = .40$, $p < .05$) but not with those of anxiety ($r_s = .21$, $p < .14$).

Study 2.   Thirty-six schizophrenic patients were followed longitudinally throughout their hospital stay with biweekly ratings. They were rated for a mean total of 13 times each, during a mean hospital stay of 6 months. Haloperidol was the only neuroleptic used, and its daily dose varied from 0 to 60 mg/day depending on the patients' clinical needs. The mean ($\pm$ SD) daily dose was 29.0 $\pm$ 31.1 mg. We compared the mean BPRS ratings for the three

Table 7 A Comparison of the Three Groups (Study 2)

	Persistent TD (N = 8)	Intermittent TD (N = 9)	Non-TD (N = 19)
Age (years)	35 ± 6	34 ± 7	31 ± 7
Gender (M/F)	3/5	6/3	9/10
Daily Dose (mg) of Haloperidol	25.7 ± 28.0	41.0 ± 29.5	24.7 ± 36.2
Simpson's TD Score (minimum 17)	28 ± 8	24 ± 6	19 ± 2
Total AIMS Score	9 ± 5	5 ± 4	1 ± 2
Total BPRS Score	13 ± 5	13 ± 6	12 ± 7

NOTE.   Values (except for gender) represent means ± SD. TD = tardive dyskinesia; AIMS = Abnormal Involuntary Movement Scale; BPRS = Brief Psychiatric Rating Scale.

Table 8 Tardive Dyskinesia (TD) and Symptoms of Schizophrenia (Study 2)

	Persistent TD (N = 8)	Intermittent TD (N = 9)	Non-TD (N = 19)
Positive Symptoms	1.3 ± 1.1	1.5 ± 0.6	1.1 ± 0.9
Negative Symptoms*	2.6 ± 1.1	2.3 ± 0.4	1.8 ± 0.8

NOTE.   Values represent means ± SD.
* $p < .05$, Duncan's Multiple Range Test.

groups and correlated them with the severity of TD as judged by the AIMS and Simpson scale at three dosage levels of haloperidol: low dose (<20 mg/day), moderate dose (20–40 mg/day), and high dose (>40 mg/day).

The persistent TD, intermittent TD, and non-TD groups did not differ from one another in terms of age, gender, daily dose of haloperidol, or mean total rating on the BPRS (Table 7). As expected, the persistent TD group had the highest and the non-TD group the lowest score on the Simpson TD scale and the AIMS. Among the individual syndromes of the BPRS, the only one that significantly differentiated the three groups was the negative symptom subscale. The persistent TD patients had the highest and the non-TD patients the lowest scores on the negative symptoms ($p < .05$, Duncan's Multiple Range test; Table 8). In both TD groups, the fluctuations in total TD scores on the Simpson scale as well as the AIMS with different dosage levels of haloperidol paralleled those on the BPRS (total and negative symptoms).

Discussion

Our cross-sectional study of neuroleptic-free patients suggested an association between TD and depressive as well as negative symptoms of schizophrenia. The longitudinal study of patients on different dosages of haloperidol confirmed the association of TD (especially persistent TD) with negative symptoms. The latter include emotional withdrawal, motor retardation, and blunted affect. It is interesting to relate our findings to the concept of the so-called subcortical dementia discussed earlier. Our patients with TD (especially persistent TD) had a movement disorder, motor retardation, and apathy. Their memory difficulty, if any, remains to be ascertained with the help of neuropsychological testing. Nevertheless, the apparent similarity with the reported subcortical dementias raises a possibility that subcortical (e.g., basal ganglia) damage might be related to certain major clinical manifestations of our persistent TD patients.

One alternative explanation for the association between persistent TD and negative symptoms is that schizophrenic patients with negative symptoms may need higher amounts of neuroleptics, resulting in the development of TD. We should add, however, that among our patients, there was no significant correlation between severity of negative symptoms and total intake of neuroleptics.

Our study does not support the notion of the supersensitivity psychosis. Chouinard and Jones (1980), who proposed the concept, reported an association between TD and positive symptoms of schizophrenia. Our findings were in the opposite direction.

We observed an association between persistent TD and depressive syndrome in our neuroleptic-free patients. This finding is consistent with the reports of a somewhat higher prevalence of TD in patients with affective disorders (see Chapter 5). It is unlikely that the patients' depression was secondary to TD, since the TD patients were significantly less anxious than the non-TD ones. There is an obvious overlap between depressive symptoms and negative symptoms of schizophrenia. Such an overlap may explain, at least partially, the higher proportion of depressed and lower proportion of anxious patients in the persistent TD group.

SUMMARY

Movement disorders tend to be associated with various psychiatric disturbances. No single pattern of psychpathology is consistently found in different movement disorders. A common form of psychopathology reported in patients with movement disorders is either apathy or depression. Varying degrees of dementia are also present in many of these patients. It is uncertain whether any associated cerebral cortical pathology can fully explain these behavioral manifestations. The possibility that subcortical damage, such as lesions of basal ganglia, may be at least partially responsible for both the movement disorder and certain disturbances of higher mental function deserves serious consideration.

References

Adams RD, Victor M: Principles of Neurology. 2nd ed. New York, McGraw-Hill, 1981

Albert ML: Subcortical dementia, in Alzheimer's Disease: Senile Dementia and Related Disorders. Edited by Terry RD, Bick KL. New York, Raven Press, 1978, pp 173–179, 194–196

Albert ML, Feldman RG, Willis AL: The "subcortical dementia" of progressive supranuclear palsy. J Neurol Neurosurg Psychiatry 37:121–130, 1974

American Psychiatric Association: Diagnostic and Statistical Manual of Mental Disorders, 3rd ed. Washington, DC, American Psychiatric Association, 1980

Benson DF: Subcortical dementia: a clinical approach, in The Dementias. Edited by Mayeux R, Rosen WG. New York, Raven Press, 1983, pp 185–194

Boller F, Mizutani T, Roessmann U, et al: Parkinson disease, dementia, and Alzheimer disease: clinicopathological correlations. Ann Neurol 7:329–335, 1980

Bolt JMW: Huntington's chorea in the west of Scotland. Br J Psychiatry 116:259–270, 1970

Bowen FP: Behavioral alterations in patients with basal ganglia lesions, in The Basal Ganglia. Edited by Yahr MD. New York, Raven Press, 1976, pp 169–180

Bowman M, Lewis MS: Sites of subcortical damage in diseases which resemble schizophrenia. Neuropsychologia 18:597–601, 1980

Brain L, Walton JN: Brain's Diseases of the Nervous System. 7th ed., New York, Oxford University Press, 1969

Brothers C: Huntington's chorea in Victoria and Tasmania. J Neurol Sci 1:405–420, 1964

Bruetsch WL: Chronic rheumatic brain disease as a possible factor in the causation of some cases of dementia praecox. Am J Psychiatry 97:276–296, 1940

Bruetsch WL: Late cerebral sequelae of rheumatic fever. Arch Intern Med 73:472–482, 1944

Caine EG, Shoulson I: Psychiatric syndromes in Huntington's disease. Am J Psychiatry 140:728–733, 1983

Carpenter MB: Human Neuroanatomy. 2nd ed. Baltimore, Williams & Wilkins, 1976, pp 496–520

Chandler JH, Reed TE, DeJong RN: Huntington's chorea in Michigan, III: clinical observations. Neurology (Minneapolis) 10:148–153, 1960

Chouinard G, Jones BD: Neuroleptic-induced supersensitivity psychosis: clinical and pharmacologic characteristics. Am J Psychiatry 137:16–21, 1980

Cutler NR, Post RM, Rey AC, et al: Depression-dependent dyskinesias in two cases of manic-depressive illness. N Engl J Med 18:1088–1089, 1981

DaMasio AR, DaMasio H, Rizzo M, et al: Aphasia with nonhemorrhagic lesions in the basal ganglia and internal capsule. Arch Neurol 39:15–20, 1982

Degkwitz R: Extrapyramidal motor disorders following long-term treatment with neuroleptic drugs, in Psychotropic Drugs and Dysfunctions of the Basal Ganglia. Edited by Crane GE, Gardner JR Jr. Washington, DC, US Government Printing Office, 1969, pp 22–32

DeReuck J, Crevits L, DeCoster W, et al: Pathogenesis of Binswanger chronic progressive subcortical encephalopathy. Neurology 30:920–928, 1980

Dewhurst K, Oliver JE, McKnight AL: Socio-psychiatric consequences of Huntington's disease. Br J Psychiatry 116:255-258, 1970

Dobyns WB, Goldstein NP, Gordon H: Clinical spectrum of Wilson's disease (hepatolenticular degeneration). Mayo Clin Proc 54:35–42, 1979

Fedio P, Cox CS, Neophytides A, et al: Neuropsychological profile of Huntington's disease: patients and those at risk, in Advances in Neurology, Vol 23: Huntington's Disease. Edited by Chase TN, Wexler NS, Barbeau A. New York, Raven Press, 1979, pp 239–255

Folstein SE, Folstein MF, McHugh PR: Psychiatric syndromes in Huntington's disease, in Advances in Neurology, Vol 23: Huntington's Disease. Edited by Chase TN, Wexler NS, Barbeau A. New York, Raven Press, 1979, pp 281–289

Freeman JM, Aron AM, Collard JE, et al: The emotional correlates of Sydenham's chorea. Pediatrics 35:42–49, 1965

Gilles de la Tourette G: Etude sur une affection nerveuse caracterisée par de l'incoordination motrice accompagnée d'echolalie et de copralalie. Arch Neurol (Paris) 9:19–42, 1885

Glazer WM, Moore DC, Schooler NR, et al: Tardive dyskinesia: a discontinuation study. Arch Gen Psychiatry 41:623–627, 1984

Graybiel AM, Ragsdale CW Jr: Fiber connections of the basal ganglia. Prog Brain Res 51:239–283, 1979

Grinber RR, Sahs AL: Neurology. 6th ed. Springfield, Charles C. Thomas, 1966

Guttman E: On some constitutional aspects of chorea and on its sequelae. J Neurol Psychopathol 17:16–26, 1936

Hamra BJ, Nasrallah HA, Clancy J, et al: Psychiatric diagnosis and tardive dyskinesia (letter to editor). Arch Gen Psychiatry 40:346–347, 1983

Healthfield KWG: Huntington's chorea. Brain 90:203–232, 1967

Hippius M, Lange J: Zur problematik der spaten extrapyramidalen hyperkinesen nach Langfristiger neuroleptischer Therapie. Arzneimittel Forschung 20:888–890, 1970

Huntington G: On chorea. Med Surg Rep 26:317–321, 1872

James W, Mefferd R, Kimbell I: Early signs of Huntington's chorea. Diseases of the Nervous System 30:558–559, 1969

Jankovic J, Ford J: Blepharospasm and orofacial-cervical dystonia: clinical and pharmacological findings in 100 patients. Ann Neurol 13:402–411, 1983

Jeste DV, Wyatt RJ: Changing epidemiology of tardive dyskinesia. Am J Psychiatry 138:297–309, 1981

Jeste DV, Wyatt RJ: Therapeutic strategies against tardive dyskinesia: two decades of experience. Arch Gen Psychiatry 39:803–816, 1982a

Jeste DV, Wyatt RJ: Understanding and Treating Tardive Dyskinesia. New York, Guilford Press, 1982b

Jeste DV, Karson CN, Iager A, et al: Association of abnormal involuntary movements and negative symptoms. Psychopharmacol Bull 1984 (in press)

Kendall BE, Pollock SS, Bass NM, et al: Wilson's disease—clinical correlation with cranial computed tomography. Neuroradiology 22:1–5, 1981

Keshavan MS, Goswamy U: Tardive dyskinesia less severe in depression (letter to editor). Br J Psychiatry 140:207–208, 1982

Lidsky TL, Weinhold PM, Levine FM: Implications of basal ganglionic dysfunction for schizophrenia. Biol Psychiatry 14:3–12, 1979

Lieberman A, Dziatolowski M, Neophytides A, et al: Dementias of Huntington's and Parkinson's disease, in Advances in Neurology, Vol 23: Huntington's Disease. Edited by Chase TN, Wexler NS, Barbeau A. New York, Raven Press, 1979, pp 273–280

Lishman WA: Organic Psychiatry. Oxford, Blackwell Scientific Publications, 1978, pp 549–557

Loizou LA, Kendall BE, Marshall J: Subcortical arteriosclerotic encephalopathy: a clinical and radiological investigation. J Neurol Neurosurg Psychiatry 44:294–304, 1981

Lyle O, Gottesman I: Premorbid psychometric indicators of the gene for Huntington's disease. J Consult Clin Psychol 45:1011–1022, 1977

Marsden CD: Blepharospasm-oromandibular dystonia syndrome (Brueghel's syndrome): a variant of adult-onset torsion dystonia? J Neurol Neurosurg Psychiatry 39:1204–1209, 1976

Marsden CD: The diagnosis of dementia, in Studies in Geriatric Psychiatry. Edited by Isaacs AD, Post F. New York, John Wiley & Sons, 1978, pp 95–118

Marsden CD: Basal ganglia disease. Lancet 2:1141–1146, 1982

Mayeux R, Stern Y: Intellectual dysfunction and dementia in Parkinson disease, in The Dementias. Edited by Mayeux R, Rosen WG. New York, Raven Press, 1983, pp 211–227

Mayeux R, Stern Y, Rosen J, et al: Depression, intellectual impairment, and Parkinson disease. Neurology 31:645–650, 1981

Mayeux R, Stern Y, Rosen J, et al: Is "subcortical dementia" a recognizable clinical entity? Ann Neurol 14:278–283, 1983

Montgomery MA, Clayton PJ, Friedhoff AJ: Psychiatric illness in Tourette syndrome patients and first-degree relatives, in Gilles de la Tourette Syndrome. Edited by Friedhoff AJ, Chase TN. New York, Raven Press, 1982, pp 335–339

Naeser MA, Alexander MP, Helm-Estabrooks N, et al: Aphasia with predominantly subcortical lesion sites: description of three capsular/putaminal aphasia syndromes. Arch Neurol 39:2–14, 1982

National Institute of Mental Health Psychopharmacology Research Branch: Abnormal Involuntary Movement Scale. ECDEU Intercom 4:3–6, 1975

Nausieda PA, Bieliauskas L-A, Bacon LD, et al: Chronic dopaminergic supersensitivity after Sydenham's chorea. Neurology 33:750–754, 1983

Nee LE, Caine ED, Polinsky RJ, et al: Gilles de la Tourette syndrome: clinical and family study of 50 cases. Ann Neurol 7:41–49, 1980

Norton JC: Patterns of neuropsychological test performance in Huntington's disease. J Nerv Ment Dis 161:276–279, 1975

Oliver JE: Huntington's chorea in Northamptonshire. Br J Psychiatry 116:241–253, 1970

Overall JE, Gorham DR: The Brief Psychiatric Rating Scale. Psychol Rep 10:799–812, 1962

Pandey RS, Sreenivas KN, Patil NM, et al: Dopamine β-hydroxylase inhibition in a patient with Wilson's disease and manic symptoms. Am J Psychiatry 138:1628–1629, 1981

Parkinson J: An essay on the shaking palsy, 1817. Med Class 2:964–997, 1938

Schwartzman J: Chorea minor: review of 175 cases with reference to etiology, treatment and sequelae. Rheumatism 6:89–95, 1950

Seigel S: Non-Parametric Statistics. New York, McGraw-Hill, 1956

Simpson GM, Angus JWS: A rating scale for extrapyramidal side effects. Acta Psychiatr Scand 212:11–19, 1970

Simpson GM, Lee JM, Zoubok B, et al: A rating scale for tardive dyskinesia. Psychopharmacology 64:171–179, 1979

Spitzer RL, Endicott J, Robins E: Research Diagnostic Criteria (RDC) for a Selected Group of Functional Disorders. 3rd ed. New York, Biometrics Research, 1977

Sroka H, Elizan TS, Yahr MD, et al: Organic mental syndrome and confusional states in Parkinson's disease. Arch Neurol 38:339–342, 1981

Stern Y: Behavior and the basal ganglia, in The Dementias. Edited by Mayeux R, Rosen WG. New York, Raven Press, 1983, pp 195–207

Stollerman GH: Rheumatic fever, in Principles of Internal Medicine. Edited by Petersdorf RG, Adams RD, Brauwald E, et al. New York, McGraw-Hill, 1983, pp 1397–1402

Teuber H-L: Complex functions of basal ganglia, in The Basal Ganglia. Edited by Yahr MD. New York, Raven Press, 1976, pp 151–168

Tolosa ES: Clinical features of Meige's disease (idiopathic orofacial dystonia): a report of 17 cases. Arch Neurol 38:147–151, 1981

Victor M: Discussion, in Alzheimer's Disease: Senile Dementia and Related Disorders. Edited by Terry RD, Bick K. New York, Raven Press, 1978, pp 194–196

Wallesch CW, Kornhuber HH, Kunz T, et al: Neuropsychological deficits associated with small unilateral thalamic lesions. Brain 106:141–152, 1983

Wexler NS: Perceptual-motor, cognitive, and emotional characteristics of persons at risk for Huntington's disease, in Advances in Neurology, Vol 23: Huntington's Disease. Edited by Chase TN, Wexler NS, Barbeau A. New York, Raven Press, 1979, pp 239–255

Whitehouse PJ, Price DL, Struble RG, et al: Alzheimer's disease and senile dementia: loss of neurons in the basal forebrain. Science 215:1237–1239, 1982

Whittier J: Hereditary chorea (Huntington's chorea): a paradigm of brain damage with psychopathology, in Psychopathology and Brain Dysfunction. Edited by Shagass C, Gershon E, Friedhoff AJ. New York, Raven Press, 1977, pp 267–277

Wilson SAK: Progressive lenticular degeneration: a familial nervous disease associated with cirrhosis of the liver. Brain 34:295–509, 1912